In-Office Lab Testing
Functional Terrain Analysis

TABLE OF CONTENTS

ACKNOWLEDGEMENTS

Many thanks to Lucinda for your support during the writing of this book. Special thanks to John Sherman, ND. Your work has inspired my exploration into terrain medicine and Functional Urinalysis.

This book has incorporated information from a variety of practitioners without prejudice to degree. We have used interpretations and concepts from Medicine, Naturopathy, Biochemistry, and Nutrition. We would specifically like to thank the following for their contributions to our understanding of Functional Diagnosis.

Lynn August, MD
Dan Carter, ND
Harry Eidenier, PhD
Patricia Kane, PhD
Harold Krystal, DDS
Harold Loomis, DC
Russell Marz, ND
Stephen Stiteler, L.Ac

Joseph Montante, MD
James Said, DC, ND
Steven Sandberg-Lewis, ND
Alexander Schauss, Ph.D.
Guy Schenker, DC
John Sherman, ND
Dickson Thom, DDS, ND
Jeffrey Bland, PhD

INTRODUCTION

The Terrain

The terrain describes the inner environment of the body. It is the regulation of pH, oxidation/reduction, mineral balance, enzyme kinetics, hormonal communication, nutrient delivery and waste removal between the extra-cellular fluids (blood, saliva, urine and lymph) and the tissues and cells of the body that co-exist and interact in these fluids. The body has an amazing capacity for self-regulation in the face of the mild stresses of everyday life. Terrain damage and the emergence of functional disturbances occurs when the self-regulatory capacities of the body are overwhelmed by increasing amounts of stressors, such as antibiotics, nutrient deficiencies, vaccinations and environmental toxins.

Symptoms, such as fatigue, low energy, reduced immunity and digestive dysfunction, are merely the expression of the terrain damage and are viewed as communication between the body and the outside world. The focus of treatment, therefore, is not to stop or suppress symptoms but instead to address the underlying imbalances.

Patients with these symptoms often present without clinical findings i.e. their blood tests, pathology reports etc. appear within "normal" range. One of the primary benefits of Functional Terrain Assessment is its ability to address subtle imbalances before severe damage sets in, bringing the body back into its normal state of equilibrium.

Functional Terrain Analysis

Functional Terrain Analysis is a systemized method of in-office testing that allows the physician to assess the self-regulatory capacities of the body. It allows the physician to do the following:

- Assess whether the inner environment of the body is in a state of balance or not.

- Identify the specific areas of imbalance.

- Address the imbalances by making appropriate therapeutic recommendations.

- Re-check to see that the body has been brought back to a state of balance after treatment.

The physician is able to make this assessment using a comprehensive series of tests that evaluate saliva and urine and other parameters for the following:

- Acid-base equilibrium in the body

- Specific mineral imbalances

- Effects of stress on the body

- Presence of abnormal metabolites in the body

- Digestion, absorption, assimilation and utilization of macro and micro nutrients

- Overgrowth of abnormal bacteria in the digestive system

- Evidence of adrenal dysfunction

- Presence of free radicals and increasing oxidative stress in the body

- Antioxidant status

Functional Terrain Analysis has the following benefits:

- Allows the practitioner to identify and address subtle imbalances before severe damage sets in

- Provides the practitioner with immediate and easily accessible in-office information to determine the imbalances in the physiology and biochemistry of the patients

- Stops the endless cycle of chasing symptoms and gets to the cause of the problem

- Serves as a teaching guide to share with the patient, thus allowing them to take a more active role in their health care

- Acts as "Gateway tests" by helping the practitioner determine the need for additional and more specific laboratory assays

- The practitioner has a clear way to document a starting point or reference point to determine if the treatment plan is working

- Does not rely on expensive equipment and lab tests

It is important to remember that the terrain assessment tests do not diagnose any specific pathology or disease states. They are prognostic signposts to help in the functional assessment of the patient.

Gastrointestinal Terrain

NOTES:

THE GASTROINTESTINAL TERRAIN

Assessing the Gastrointestinal Terrain

The state of the gastrointestinal terrain can be assessed using the following tests:

1. Gastrotest for stomach pH.

2. Bowel Toxicity Test (Urinary indican test)

3. Urinary Sediment Test

4. Urine Calcium

5. Urine Specific Gravity

Disturbances to the Gastrointestinal Terrain

These tests can be used to detect the presence of the following functional disturbances to the gastrointestinal terrain:

1. Dysbiosis

2. Bowel toxemia

3. Pancreatic insufficiency

4. Hypochlorhydria

5. Malabsorption

6. Leaky gut syndrome

DYSBIOSIS

-   The GI tract is an ecosystem, with a balance between aerobic and anaerobic microorganisms.

-   It has been estimated that there are over 500 species of bacteria and there are many more bacterial cells in the intestines than there are in the whole body.

NOTES:

- The majority of the bacteria are located in the colon. In a healthy gut the dominant flora is composed of beneficial bacteria of the Lactobacillus and Bifidobacteria species.

Functions of beneficial bacteria

1. Produce vitamins such as folic acid and B12.

2. Nourish the lining of the colon by feeding on vegetable fiber and producing butyric acid. Adequate butyric acid levels reduce the chances for colon cancer.

3. Inhibit harmful bacteria.

4. Break down toxins.

Dysbiosis as a cause of terrain imbalance

Dysbiosis is the overgrowth of harmful bacteria that causes disease. It can exist in the oral cavity, the gastrointestinal system or vaginal cavity. In gastrointestinal dysbiosis, organisms such as yeast, bacteria and parasites induce disease in the following ways:

- Inhibit normal bacteria, creating deficiencies of nutrients and other problems.

- Cause inflammation in the digestive system compromising absorption and contributing to deficiencies of nutrients, proteins, carbohydrates and fats

- Produce toxins. Harmful bacteria create toxins and inhibit normal bacteria from detoxifying the bowel. Toxins can burden the liver and the body's detoxification system affecting every function in the body.

- Lower the levels of short chain fatty acids, thus increasing the risk of colon cancer and ulcerative colitis

- Hydrogenate polyunsaturated fatty acids

- Irritate the lining of the intestine, increasing intestinal permeability (leaky gut).

Some of the common causes of dysbiosis include:

1. Antibiotic therapy

2. Hypochlorhydria

3. Presence of xenobiotics such as chemicals and heavy metals

NOTES:

4.   Exposure to pathogens/parasitic infections

5.   Pancreatic insufficiency

6.   Slow bowel transit time/bowel stasis

7.   Poor immune function and low intestinal secretory IgA

8.   Nutrient deficiencies

9.   A fiber deficient diet

10.   Increased intestinal pH

Dysbiosis has been associated with the following diseases and disorders:

- Chronic gastrointestinal problems e.g. Irritable bowel syndrome and Inflammatory Bowel Disease

- Inflammatory or autoimmune disorders such as ankylosing spondylitis, fibromyalgia and arthritis

- Food allergy and intolerance,

- Breast and colon cancer

- Unexplained fatigue

- Malnutrition

- Atopic eczema

- Pancreatic insufficiency

- Intestinal hyperpermeability

- Candidiasis

NOTES:

BOWEL TOXEMIA

- Bowel toxemia is the excessive production of toxic metabolites of digestion especially in the colon.

- The liver detoxifies toxins produced by the gut. If the liver is not functioning optimally or if the amount of toxin production overwhelms its metabolic capabilities, the toxins can enter the systemic circulation and cause numerous health problems.

Intestinal toxins and the diseases/conditions they are associated with:

1. **Histamine:** headaches, arrhythmias, depression, low blood pressure, nausea

2. Putricene and cadaverine: low blood pressure

3. **Ammonia:** coma, tremors, altered EEG, mental changes

4. Indole (from Tryptophan): bladder tumors

5. **Phenol:** depressed CNS and circulation, mucosal irritation, damage to kidney and liver

6. **Skatole (from Tryptophan):** injures red blood cells and hemoglobin molecules, depressed CNS and circulation

7. **Hydrogen sulfide (from protein breakdown):** mucosal irritation, congestion and increased intestinal permeability; depressed CNS and circulation

Some of the causes of bowel toxemia include the following:

- Poor digestion

- Slow peristalsis, slow bowel transit time or bowel sluggishness

- Constipation

- Exposure to excessive chemicals in the water, food, air, and drugs

- Abnormal bowel flora: yeast/candida, parasites or bacteria

NOTES:

Some of the signs and symptoms of bowel toxemia include:

- Gas

- Diarrhea

- Constipation

- Bad breath

- Bloating

- Weight gain

- Allergies

- Asthma

- Arthritis

- Headaches

- Skin conditions

- Nervous system problems

- Colon toxicity which is directly associated with low back pain and sciatica.

Bowel toxemia is associated with the following conditions:

- Maldigestion

- Flatulence

- Irregular stools

- Psoriasis

- Acne

- Eczema

- Fatigue

NOTES:

PANCREATIC INSUFFICIENCY

Pancreatic insufficiency is a condition of decreased output of pancreatic enzymes, such as lipase, amylase, cellulase and protease, into the small intestine.

The net effect is a failure to obtain optimal nourishment from the breakdown of proteins, carbohydrates, fats and fiber.

Common causes of pancreatic insufficiency

1. Overeating, which can exhaust the pancreatic enzyme output

2. A diet high in cooked foods that rely too heavily on pancreatic enzymes.

3. Eating too many devitalized foods lacking zinc, manganese, vitamin B6 and magnesium, which are all vital minerals for optimum pancreatic enzyme function.

4. Insufficient protein, which will not provide the pancreas the amino acids needed for creating enzymes

5. A diet that is deficient in fiber and too high in refined sugar.

6. Systemic acidosis. The body will try to conserve the bicarbonate produced by the pancreas to help reverse the acidosis.

7. A spasm in the duodenum can cut off the supply of bicarbonate

Some of the signs and symptoms of Pancreatic insufficiency include:

1. Steatorrhea (greasy, fatty, floating stools)

2. Diarrhea

3. Maldigestion

4. Stools with a lot of undigested food

5. Acne

6. Food allergies

7. Hypoglycemic symptoms

NOTES:

8. Abnormal weight gain, or more commonly, weight loss

HYPOCHLORHYDRIA

Hypochlorhydria is a condition of decreased secretions of hydrochloric acid and pepsin from the parietal cells in the stomach.

It is a condition generally associated with aging but can affect anyone at any age.

Common causes of hypochlorhydria

1. Autoimmune diseases (anti-parietal cell antibody)

2. Helicobacter pylori infection

3. Antacid drugs such as Tagamet, Prilosec, Xantac and Pepcid AC

4. Chronic eating of devitalized food

5. Excess dietary fat, sugar, alcohol, caffeine and refined foods

6. Chronic overeating can "exhaust" the stomach, which has to concentrate the hydrogen ion by 4 million times than in arterial blood

7. Hypothyroidism

8. Hypoadrenalism

9. Chronic stress

10. Recurrent food poisoning or excessive dysbiosis (bacterial, parasitic, yeast, fungal)

11. Excess carbohydrate consumption, as in a vegan diet

12. The effects of low stomach acid can be insidious and progressive.

Signs and symptoms of hypochlorhydria

- Bloating, belching, burning and flatulence after a meal

- A sense of fullness after a meal

- Indigestion, diarrhea and constipation, Undigested food in the stool

NOTES:

- Nausea after taking supplements

- Rectal itching

- Weak, peeling or cracked nails

- Dilated capillaries in cheeks and nose in non-alcoholics

- Post adolescent acne

- Iron deficiency

- Chronic intestinal infections and dysbiosis

Diseases and disorders linked with hypochlorhydria

1. Diabetes mellitus

2. Childhood asthma

3. Thryroid: hypothyroid, hyperthyroid

4. Skin: eczema, vitiligo, rosacea, psoriasis

5. Gall bladder disease: cholelithiasis, cholecystitis

6. Hepatitis

7. Osteoporosis

8. Chronic autoimmune disorders: Rheumatoid arthritis, Lupus erythematosus

9. Urticaria

10. Adrenal exhaustion

11. Chronic atrophic gastritis

MALABSORPTION

Malabsorption is the inability of nutrients to be absorbed through the intestinal mucosal cells. It is characterized by the abnormal excretion of fat in the stool (steatorrhea) and the malabsorption of proteins, carbohydrates, fats, minerals and vitamins.

NOTES:

It is possible to have a malabsorption of one nutrient but not any of the others because they may all be absorbed by different processes. It is also possible to have malabsorption and leaky gut syndrome at the same time

Common causes of malabsorption

1. Inadequate fat emulsification due to insufficient bile salts

2. Enzyme deficiency causing defective protein, fat or carbohydrate breakdown

3. Diarrhea or a decreased bowel transit time, which does not allow for optimal absorption

4. Abnormalities with the cell membrane

5. Decreased surface area of the intestinal lumen (celiac disease)

6. Intestinal infection

Diseases closely associated with malabsorption

*   Celiac disease

*   Crohn's disease

*   Giardiasis

*   Lactose intolerance

LEAKY GUT SYNDROME

The small intestine functions as a permeable barrier.

On the one hand it is an absorptive organ with the active and passive movement of nutrients through the cell and on the other hand serves as a barrier to toxic compounds and large molecules, which are prevented from entering the blood stream by tight junctions between the intestinal mucosal cells.

Damage to the intestinal mucosa and the tight junctions can lead to a hyper permeable intestinal lumen, causing leaky gut syndrome. The symptoms of leaky gut syndrome result from increased permeability of large macromolecules including dietary and microbial polypeptides and polysaccharides.

NOTES:

Bacterial endotoxins, food allergens, and even viable bacteria can penetrate the intestinal mucosa, causing local and systemic inflammation, and if they get into the bloodstream induce antibody reactions with host tissues and form immune complexes.

Causes of Leaky gut syndrome or Intestinal hyperpermeability

1. Parasitic infections: giardiasis

2. Excessive use of Non Steroidal Anti-inflammatory Drugs (aspirin, etc.)

3. Maldigestion/malabsorption

4. Intestinal dysbiosis

5. Deficient secretory IgA

6. Pancreatic insufficiency

7. Excessive use of alcohol.

Disorders associated with Leaky gut syndrome

- Inflammatory bowel disease

- Crohn's disease

- Inflammatory joint disease

- Celiac disease

- Food allergies

- Auto-immune diseases: ankylosing spondylitis, rheumatoid arthritis

- HIV infection and AIDS

NOTES:

Tests to Assess Gastrointestinal Functional Disturbances

- Bowel Toxicity test
- Urine sediment test
- Urine calcium test
- Urine Specific Gravity
- Gastro-Test for stomach pH

You can make clinical assessments by either looking at the tests individually or by observing the patterns between two or more tests. The section on patterns, in the back of the manual, will give you more detailed information. The following section will present each of these tests individually.

NOTES:

GASTRO-TEST (GASTRIC STRING TEST)

Discussion

 The Gastro-test is a very safe and effective method of assessing stomach pH.

The Gastro-Test itself is 70cm of a highly absorbent cotton string coiled inside a weighted gelatin capsule.

The capsule is swallowed and retrieved from the stomach after 10 minutes. The string is rubbed with a pH stick and the color obtained compared to a pH chart provided with each capsule.

The Gastro-test is a test that can be used to check for both for ambient stomach pH and the body's ability to respond to a challenge.

When would you run this test?

- To check a patient's stomach pH for evidence of hypochlorhydria and to see whether the stomach can produce acid in response to a challenge

Directions

1. Have patient eat a protein rich meal 2 hours before test.

2. For an ambient pH have patient fast for 8-10 hours.

3. Get patient to swallow a little water to lubricate the throat

4. Swallow the capsule with a little water while the free end is held firmly outside the mouth

5. After capsule has been swallowed patient lies on left side or back on the table for 10 minutes.

6. After 10 minutes get the patient to sit up and with chin raised swiftly remove the string.

7. Lay string on paper and while the string is still moist touch the pH stick to the string starting at the distal end

8. The resultant colors are compared with the pH chart that comes with the test

9. Discoloration of any segment of the string represents acid pooling

NOTES:

10. Do not expect the whole string to be a consistent color

NOTE: be aware that the string is contaminated with stomach juices and can therefore contain Helicobacter pylori bacteria and even parasitic residue.

Use the following information if patient's have a high pH reading with the Gastro-test.

Results

1. Any result of pH 3 or lower indicates the stomach is able to secrete acid normally.

2. If stomach pH is above pH 3, follow the directions below by dynamically assessing the stomach's ability to secrete stomach acid after a challenge with sodium bicarbonate or stimulation with secretagogues, such as bitter herbs or caffeine

Direction for bicarbonate challenge or secretagogue stimulation

Stimulation	Bicarbonate Challenge
• A patient can have their ambient stomach pH taken after an 8-10 hour fast. • There should be an acidic pH, even on a fasting test • If the result shows a more alkaline pH, you can see whether or not the parietal cells can produce stomach acid in response stimulation by bitters such as gentian and scutellaria or caffeine, which all cause the secretion of stomach acid. • The stomach should acidify after a stimulation	• A patient can be checked after eating a high protein meal, which should cause adequate acidification in the stomach. • If the patient's stomach pH is alkaline after the Gastro-test, you can see whether or not the parietal cells can produce stomach acid in response to an alkaline challenge (sodium bicarbonate). • The stomach should produce stomach acid and acidify after such a challenge

NOTES:

RESULTS
<ul><li>If after the initial test the stomach pH is above pH_3, redo the test 30 minutes after stimulation with bitter herbs, such as gentian/scutellaria (use 4 capsules as a challenge), or caffeine, in the form of a standardized dose (No-Doze) (use 1 standardized tablet)</li> <li>The stomach should be in the normal range after 30 minutes</li> <li>If after stimulation the stomach pH remains 5 or above, achlorhydria presumably exists.</li> <li>Consistent low pH after fasting indicates dysfunctional timing of stomach acid secretion.</li></ul>	<ul><li>If after the initial test the stomach pH is above pH3, redo the test 30 minutes after stimulation with a sodium bicarbonate drink (1 teaspoon dissolved in ¼ cup of water)</li> <li>The stomach should be in the normal range after 30 minutes</li> <li>If after stimulation the stomach pH remains 5 or above, achlorhydria presumably exists.</li></ul>

NOTES:

Clinical implications

High stomach pH

Clinical Implication	Additional information
Hypochlorhydria	Re-do the test after a bicarbonate challenge or stimulation with bitters or caffeine to see if the body can respond to the challenge by producing HCl
Achlorhydria	Stomach pH remains above 5.0 after challenge with bicarbonate or bitters

Low stomach pH

Clinical Implication	Additional information
Dysfunctional timing	If the ambient fasting stomach pH is consistently low consider that the timing of stomach acid secretions is abnormal i.e. the stomach is trickling stomach acid out even when there is not a stimulus for its production.
Hypersecretion of acid	In our experience the hypersecretion of stomach acid is quite rare and is usually a problem of dysfunctional timing than a pure hyper secretion of acid.

Related Tests

- Urinary Indican,

- Heidelberg Test

- Helicobacter pylori Testing

- Blood Chemistry evaluation of hypochlorhydria (See our book entitled "Blood Chemistry and CBC Analysis- Clinical Laboratory Testing from a Functional Perspective" for more details.)

- Urine Sediment Testing

NOTES:

BOWEL TOXICITY TEST (URINE INDICAN TEST, OBERMEYER'S TEST)

Discussion

 A group of toxic phenolic compounds (indol, putricene, cadavorene and other putrefying gases) are produced from the putrification of partially digested food by an overgrowth of unfriendly anaerobic bacteria in the small and large intestine.

Indican is formed when anaerobic intestinal bacteria converts the amino acid Tryptophan into indole.

The indole is absorbed into the blood stream and is converted into indican or 3-hydroxy indole in the liver, combined with potassium sulfate and glucoronic acid, then returned to the blood and excreted by the kidneys.

The presence of indican in the urine is a sign of the following:

1. Putrification in the gut,

2. A lack of normal bowel flora (lactobacillus)

3. Excessive free oil consumption in a fat-intolerant person

Elevated levels of indican are an indication of the following:

*   Hypochlorhydria

*   Bowel toxemia

*   Protein maldigestion

*   Bad food combining

*   Slow transit time

*   Dysbiosis

*   A failure to emulsify fats and possible candidiasis.

NOTES:

The higher the level of indican the greater the degree of constipation and/or diarrhea, lower bowel gas and the greater the need for colon cleansing and digestive support.

When would you run this test?

1. To evaluate digestive function

2. To assess for dysbiosis

3. To evaluate bowel toxicity

The testing uses the following reagents:

1. Obermeyer's reagent
2. Chloroform
3. Potassium chlorate

NOTE: Obermeyer's reagent is a strong acid that will cause burns. Wear safety goggles, rubber gloves and protective clothing.

A few words of caution about Obermeyer's reagent and the Bowel Toxicty Test:

- Do not pour the reagents from the Bowel Toxicity Test down your sink. The acid in the Obermeyer's reagent will quickly damage your plumbing. I suggest that you pour the reagents into the bowl of your toilet and flush.

- You do not need a hooded vent to do the Bowel toxicity test. I highly recommend safety glasses, and of course gloves. Do this test in a well ventilated space, preferably with a extraction fan.

- Do not store your Obermeyer's reagent in a cabinet with metal hinges. The acid in the reagent can corrode the metal hinges over time. I found out about this the hard way!

Directions

It is best to use the first morning urine sample, which gives the most information on cellular metabolism and is a reflection of liver activity.

1. Pour 5ml of urine into a 15ml graduated centrifuge test tube

2. Add 5ml of Obermeyer's reagent

NOTES:

3. Seal the graduated centrifuge tube with parafilm, hold in place with thumb and completely INVERT the tube 8 times to mix

4. Let the test tube sit for at least 5 minutes or until cool

5. Remove parafilm and add 2 ml of chloroform

6. Place a finger cot on a thumb and mix solution by inverting 8 times

7. Allow the chloroform to settle to the bottom.

8. Examine the color in the chloroform layer. A blue color indicates the presence of indican.

9. If the chloroform remains colorless, record "Zero" in the urinalysis report form.

10. If chloroform is blue add the saturated potassium chlorate solution, a drop at a time, mixing twice after each addition, and record the number of drops necessary to decolorize the chloroform.

11. Record the number of drops of potassium chlorate used to decolorize the blue in the urinalysis report form.

NOTES:

Results

Increasing numbers of drops needed to decolorize the chloroform is an indication of increased indican levels and therefore increasing putrification in the gut.

# of Drops		Result
0	**Normal**	There should be no indican in the urine
1-3	**Mild**	Beginnings of mild dysbiosis and toxemia Possible functional hypochlorhydria
4-7	**Moderate**	Functional hypochlorhydria, heavy dysbiosis and leaky gut syndrome are likely
>7	**Severe**	Severe dysbiosis, leaky gut and malabsorption Run digestive stool analysis to further assess digestive function

Urine Indican test is a gateway test. A result of 7 or more requires further evaluation of the digestive system with a digestive stool analysis.

Clinical implications

HIGH

Clinical Implication	Additional information
Bowel toxemia	Bowel toxemia can present with the following symptoms: gas, diarrhea, constipation, bad breath, bloating, weight gain, allergies, asthma, arthritis, headaches, skin conditions, nervous system problems, and colon toxicity which are directly associated with low back pain and sciatica.
Dysbiosis	A positive test indicates dysbiosis i.e. an overgrowth of abnormal bacteria or yeast

NOTES:

Hypochlorhydria	Low levels of stomach acid can lead to the incomplete breakdown of proteins, forming the substrate for bacterial putrification and increased indican levels
Maldigestion (especially protein and fat maldigestion)	An increase in indican suggests the following: Protein is being poorly digested Protein and refined carbohydrates are being consumed at the same meal (i.e. bad food combining), A fat intolerant person is consuming excessive free oil. A failure to emulsify free oils consumed with food.
Malabsorption	Especially indicates protein malabsorption
High protein intake	Increased protein intake can overwhelm the ability of the body to digest it leaving increased levels of a substrate for bacterial putrification
Other conditions associated with increased indican include:	Ileocecal incompetence, pancreatic enzyme insufficiency, decreased peristalsis, celiac disease, halitosis, skin problems, hiatal hernia inflammatory bowel, food allergy, gastric ulcer, biliary and intestinal obstruction, Jejunal diverticulosis, Scleroderma, Postgastrectomy, Hartnup's disease,

Interfering Factors

High doses of amino acids especially tryptophan can alter the results.

Related Tests

- Digestive stool analysis

- Gastric acid assessment with Gastrotest

- Urine sediment test

- Urine calcium test

NOTES:

URINE SEDIMENT TEST

Background

The Improper digestion of the three macronutrients fats, proteins and carbohydrates can lead to dissolved sediment in the urine. The Urine sediment test causes this dissolved sediment to precipitate out, allowing you to measure the total sediment and then work out its constituents.

Discussion

Each macronutrient has very specific sediments:

1.   Carbohydrate has a sediment of calcium phosphate

2.   Protein has a sediment of Uric acid

3.   Fat has a sediment of Calcium oxalate

The urine sediment test uses a series of reagents that can determine the ratios of these sediments.

Each reagent dissolves away a specific sediment so that its level can be calculated. A first morning urine sample should have about 0.5 ml of calcium phosphate sediment, the ash resulting from the proper digestion, absorption and assimilation of carbohydrate metabolism.

Malabsorption, decreased cell permeability and sugar intolerance reduce the calcium phosphate sediment, sometimes to zero.

High total sediment indicates:

1.   Poor use (assimilation) of food,

2.   Pancreatic insufficiency,

3.   Leaky gut syndrome, all of which can lead to nutrient deficiencies as well as fat intolerance and protein maldigestion.

4.   The presence of oxalates and uric acid sediments, in addition to the phosphates normally present, indicates fat intolerance and protein maldigestion.

NOTES:

The urine sediment test is also a reflection of a patient's dietary intake. It can be used to monitor a diet diary or a dietary protocol. It will show what foods your patients have been eating and how well they are digesting.

NOTE – Check Results Against Urine Specific Gravity:

- The concentration of the urine can lead to abnormally high or abnormally low sediment.

- Check the results against the urine specific gravity.

- If the specific gravity is very high i.e. 1.025 and there is a large sediment, consider that the sediment may be unusually high due to a concentrated urine and possible dehydration.

- If the specific gravity is very low i.e. 1.005 and there is little to no sediment, consider that the sediment may be unusually low due to a dilute urine or excess water intake.

Urine sediment test and Blood Chemistry Screens

- Abnormal amounts of uric acid or calcium oxalate sediment correlate well with Blood chemistry screen values.

- Uric acid sediment is associated with an increase in serum BUN (>16mg/dL or 5.71 mmol/L), which may be elevated in kidney and liver dysfunction, hypochlorhydria or high protein intake, and an increase in serum uric acid (> 5.9 mg/dl, or 351 μmol/L), which is associated with arthralgias, chronic inflammation, oxidative stress, renal insufficiency, and leaky gut syndrome.

- Calcium oxalate is associated with an increase in serum triglycerides (>110 mg/dL or 1.24 mmol/L) and total cholesterol (>220 mg/dL or 5.69 mmol/L), which are associated with blood sugar dysregulation, liver/gallbladder dysfunction, atherosclerotic development, and low thyroid and adrenal function.

- For more information on this kind of Blood Chemistry Interpretation please see my book entitled "Blood Chemistry and CBC Analysis- Clinical Laboratory Testing from a Functional Perspective".

<u>When would you run this test?</u>

1. To determine the specific macronutrient that is being poorly digested

2. To determine type of digestive enzyme needed

3. To check for malabsorption, leaky gut syndrome and macronutrient metabolism

NOTES:

4. To assess for pancreatic insufficiency

5. To check diet diaries and patient's dietary intake

Directions

It is best to use the first morning urine sample, which gives the most information on cellular metabolism and is a reflection of liver activity.

The testing uses the following reagents:

1. 50% Ferric Nitrate

2. 10% Acetic Acid

3. 10% Sodium Hydroxide

You will need a centrifuge.

To Determine the Total Urine Sediment:

CAUTION: Ferric Nitrate will stain yellow. Avoid contact with eyes, skin and clothing

Add 10 ml of urine to a 15ml graduated centrifuge tube

1. Add 4 drops of 50% **Ferric Nitrate** solution. DO NOT shake or mix

2. Centrifuge the tube for 30 seconds

3. Pour off the fluid away from the plug of solid matter.

4. Use the wooden end of a cotton applicator stick to level the sediment in the centrifuge tube.

5. Measure the amount (volume) of sediment in ml by visualizing where the sediment would level out rather than averaging the high and low points

6. Record as total volume of the sediment on the Functional Terrain Assessment Results form.

NOTES:

To Determine Individual sediment content:

Calcium phosphate sediment:

1. Add enough **10% Acetic Acid** to equal the amount of sediment and or stir.

2. Fill to 10 ml with Distilled Water.

3. Centrifuge tube at 3400 rpm for 30 seconds.

4. If sediment completely dissolves, record 100% **Calcium Phosphate**.

5. If sediment does not completely dissolve, pour off the fluid.

6. Measure the remaining sediment.

7. Subtract the remaining sediment measurement from the total sediment recorded above and record this number (in ml) as <u>**Calcium Phosphate:**</u>

Total sediment – remaining sediment = Calcium phosphate

Uric Acid Sediment:

1. Add enough **10% Sodium Hydroxide** to equal the amount of sediment remaining in the test tube—stir well until color turns red.

2. Fill to 10 ml with Distilled Water.

3. Centrifuge the tube for 30 seconds.

4. If sediment completely dissolves—record this remainder as **Uric Acid.**

5. If sediment does not completely dissolve, pour off the fluid.

6. Measure the remaining sediment.

7. Subtract the remaining sediment from the previous remaining sediment calculated above and record this number (in ml) as <u>**Uric Acid.**</u>

Calcium Oxalate sediment:

1. Record the sediment remaining in the test tube as <u>**Calcium Oxalate**</u>.

NOTES:

Normal Values

0.5 ml of total sediment is normal

Calcium phosphate (carbohydrate sediment): 0.5ml

Uric acid (protein sediment): 0ml

Calcium oxalate (fat sediment): 0ml

Clinical implications

HIGH

Increased Calcium Phosphate

Clinical Implication	Additional information
Carbohydrate, starch and sugar maldigestion	Calcium phosphate is the sediment ash of carbohydrate metabolism. This is normally the only sediment in the urine. Increased levels can be due to a number of possible factors: 1. Deficiency in amylase enzymes. 2. Excessive simple or refined carbohydrates 3. Inability to properly metabolize simple or complex carbohydrates

Increased Uric Acid

Clinical Implication	Additional information
Protease deficiency	Uric acid is the sediment ash of improper protein metabolism. Increased levels indicate poor digestion of protein. Patients with high uric acid sediments have a tendency towards: • Loss of muscle mass
Hypochlorhydria	
Protein maldigestion	

NOTES:

Excessive protein intake	<ul><li>Poor recovery time after exercise</li><li>Hypoglycemia, sugar cravings</li><li>Poor utilization of calcium/magnesium (need specific amino acids for proper assimilation)</li></ul>

Increased Calcium oxalate

Clinical Implication	Additional information
Fat maldigestion	Calcium oxalate is the sediment ash of improper fat metabolism. Increased levels indicate poor assimilation of fats.
Lipase deficiency	
Poor fat emulsification	Patients with high calcium oxalate sediments have a tendency towards:
Calcium and magnesium deficiency	<ul><li>High cholesterol and triglycerides</li><li>Difficulty losing weight</li><li>Diabetes and cardiovascular disease.</li></ul>

NOTES:

LOW

Decreased Total Sediment or decreased Calcium phosphate sediment

Malabsorption	Low sediment levels indicate that nutrients are not crossing the gut wall, and the patient is suffering from malabsorption and decreased cell permeability. This may also be a sign of sugar intolerance.

Interfering Factors:

Falsely increased levels	Falsely decreased levels
• **Calcium oxalate-** coffee, tea, cola, chocolate and Vitamin C	• Patients who drink large amounts of water may dilute their urine to the point that little or no sediment precipitates

Related Tests

1. Bowel toxicity test,

2. Intestinal permeability studies (Lactulose/mannitol ratio),

3. Blood chemistry studies (BUN, Uric acid, Triglycerides, and Total cholesterol). Please see our book entitled "Blood Chemistry and CBC Analysis- Clinical Laboratory Testing from a Functional Perspective" for more details.

NOTES:

URINE CALCIUM (SULKOWITCH TEST)

Background

The urine calcium or Sulkowitch test is a simple test to determine the amount of calcium in the blood by testing for calcium in the urine. The test measures calcium being excreted from the body. Calcium absorption depends on the acidity of the stomach, as well as a number of other co-factors including the amount of phosphate present, and takes place in the upper small intestine.

Discussion

 The kidneys have a calcium threshold, not unlike its glucose threshold. When calcium levels in the serum rise above a certain level, it will spill into the urine. Conversely, when the serum level of calcium drops there will be no spill-over.

The kidney's serum calcium threshold is 7.5 – 9.0 mg/dL or 1.875 – 2.25 mmol/L.

The optimal serum calcium level is 9.2 – 10.0 mg/dL or 2.30 – 2.50 mmol/L, which is a value above the normal calcium threshold for the kidney. Hence, in a normal person there is usually a slight spill-over of calcium from the serum into the urine.

When the blood calcium drops below 7.5 mg/dL or 1.875 mmol/L there will be no calcium spill-over into the urine.

When the blood calcium increases above 10.0 mg/dL or 2.50 mmol/L there will be a measurable increase in calcium spill-over in the urine. The amount of calcium in the urine will also be affected by dietary intake of calcium. People on a low calcium diet may have abnormally low urine calcium.

The test can be a marker for adequate digestion and absorption. Eliminating refined foods, optimizing digestion (especially stomach pH and adequate protein digestion), and balancing the systemic pH of the body will help maintain adequate calcium levels.

Please see the section on the Tissue Mineral Assessment tests for ways to balance minerals and electrolytes.

NOTES:

When would you run this test?

1. To assess serum calcium levels.

2. As a marker for adequate digestion and absorption.

3. To monitor calcium supplementation for adequate digestion and absorption.

Directions

1. Put a dropper full of urine into a test tube

2. Add one dropper of Sulkowitch Reagent- shake to mix

3. Wait 60 seconds and observe turbidity

Results

Low calcium:	Clear:	**Little to no discernible fine white precipitate can be seen**
	Light turbidity:	**Black type can be seen and read through the test tube**
Normal:	Some turbidity:	**Black type can be seen but not read through test tube.**
High calcium:	Heavy turbidity:	**Black type cannot be seen through the test tube**
	Milky:	**It looks like milk which has been diluted with water**

NOTES:

Clinical implications

HIGH CALCIUM LEVELS

Increased urine calcium levels almost always accompany ↑ blood calcium levels

Clinical Implication	Additional information
Excess calcium consumption or supplementation	More calcium than is needed may appear in the urine causing a heavy precipitate
Excess calcium being mobilized from the bone	↑ acidosis in the body, osteoporosis, metastatic cancer, myeloma with bone metastasis, increased tissue acidosis
A diet high in refined sugars	A fast food diet high in refined carbohydrates and sugars can cause urinary calcium loss.
Thyroid hypofunction	Serum calcium may be increased in either primary thyroid hypofunction or secondary thyroid hypofunction due to anterior pituitary dysfunction. Increased serum calcium may increase the urine calcium level in this situation.
Conditions associated with an increase urine calcium	<ul><li>Parathyroid hyperfunction</li><li>Sarcoidosis</li><li>Primary cancers of the breast and bladder</li><li>Metastatic malignancies</li><li>Wilson's disease</li><li>Renal tubular acidosis</li><li>Glucocorticoid excess</li><li>Respiratory disease</li></ul>

NOTES:

LOW CALCIUM LEVELS

A low urine calcium with a clear solution indicates a low serum calcium

Clinical Implication	Additional information
Calcium need and/or a need for its co-factors	Factors that enhance calcium digestion, absorption and metabolism may need to be assessed in order to increase the urine calcium into normal range. This is especially the case with a normal urine pH. Use the Tissue mineral assessment test to fine-tune calcium and co-factor supplementation.
Hypochlorhydria	The body is unable to digest the ingested or supplemented calcium.
Excess protein intake	A very high protein diet can cause a decreased urine calcium especially with a decreased urine pH.
Malabsorption	Due to calcium's effect on the drawing of fats through the intestinal wall and protein absorption. Also celiac's disease.
Conditions associated with an decrease urine calcium	• Hypoparathyroidism • Vitamin D insufficiency • Muscle spasms • Ingestion of alkaline supplements and antacids

Interfering Factors:

Falsely increased levels	Falsely decreased levels
• Excess milk intake • Drugs: growth hormone, PTH, Vit. D • Urine taken after a high calcium meal • Corticosteroids	• Increased phosphate or bicarbonate • Antacid use • Alkaline urine • Thiazide diuretics

NOTES:

Related Tests:

1. Additional diagnostic information can be obtained by looking at urine calcium patterns with urinary pH. Please see the section of Urinary patterns for a more detailed description of patterns seen with Urine calcium.

2. Tissue mineral assessment.

3. Blood chemistry analysis of serum calcium. Please see our book entitled "Blood Chemistry and CBC Analysis- Clinical Laboratory Testing from a Functional Perspective" for more details.

NOTES:

URINE SPECIFIC GRAVITY (S.G.)

Discussion

 Specific gravity is a measurement of the total amount of material dissolved in the urine. It measures the kidney's ability to concentrate the urine.

The test is compared to the specific gravity of distilled water, which having no dissolved solutes is given the value of 1.000.

Urine has dissolved minerals and dissolved solutes of digestive residue (see Urine Sediment Test) and therefore has values above 1.000. The range of the specific gravity varies across the day due to the solids in the urine, nitrogen waste products (creatinine, urea), and the volume of fluid.

Concentrated urine with low volume will have a higher specific gravity.

Less concentrated urine with higher volume will have a lower specific gravity.

Loss of the concentrating ability of the kidneys will be reflected in the specific gravity and is an indication of renal dysfunction. The first morning specimen usually has the highest reading due to the concentrated nature of the urine, which reflects overall digestive metabolism.

Specific gravity is influenced by electrolytes, nitrogen waste products (urea, creatinine and glucose) and the metabolites formed from the incomplete digestion of macronutrients.

The urine reagent dipstick allows a basic measurement of specific gravity. We recommend that you use a urinometer to make a more accurate determination.

When would you run this test?

1. To assess the kidneys ability to concentrate the urine
2. Along with Urine adrenal test (urine chloride) to assess macronutrient digestion

Directions

Using a hydrometer will give a more accurate reading of specific gravity, than relying on the urine dipstick.

NOTES:

1. Fill urinometer with urine

2. Spin hydrometer in the urine

3. With hydrometer at eye level, read the specific gravity on the hydrometer by reading the bottom of the meniscus.

Ranges

Normal Value:	High value:	Low value:
1.010 – 1.020	> 1.020	< 1.010

Clinical implications

HIGH (concentrated urine)

Clinical Implication	Additional information
Abnormal solutes in urine	An ↑ S.G. with ↑ or normal urine volume. Need to check dipstick to confirm presence of protein or glucose.
Adrenal insufficiency	A high urinary chloride (1-13 drops of reagent) and a high specific gravity is an indication of adrenal insufficiency.
Increased mineral loss	A high specific gravity may be due to increased mineral solutes in the urine.
Digestive deficiency	An inability to properly breakdown macronutrients will lead to an increase in dissolved solutes in the urine, causing an increased specific gravity
Diabetes mellitus	Large amounts of glucose or protein ↑ the S.G. to > 1.050. Note: Every 1% of glucose in the urine will ↑ the S.G. 0.004
Dehydration	Excess water loss from sweating, fever, vomiting
Other causes of S.G. increase	Hepatic disease, Congestive heart failure, Protein malnutrition, collagen vascular disease

NOTES:

LOW (dilute urine)

Clinical Implication	Additional information
Congested lymphatic system	↓ S.G. and ↓ or normal urine volume indicates the kidney is having difficulty concentrating the urine and cleansing the blood due to a congested lymphatic system which can cause: swollen glands, allergy symptoms, low back pain, headaches and nausea. Symptoms worsen in women during menses and pregnancy, and may lead to vomiting.
Early chronic renal dz.	↓ S.G. and ↑ volume
Diabetes insipidus	↓ S.G. and ↑↑ volume
Kidney inflammation and infection	↓ S.G. and ↓ volume Glomerulonephritis (inflammation without infection) Pyelonephritis (inflammation with infection)

Interfering Factors

Falsely increased levels	Falsely decreased levels
• Excess mineral consumption • Cold urine • Moderate protein in urine • Detergent residue on specimen containers	• Specific gravity declines progressively after middle age • Highly buffered alkaline urine (dipstick only)

Related Tests

- Urine adrenal test
- Urine volume
- Urine glucose
- Urine protein
- Urine Sediment Test

Minerals and
Electrolytes

NOTES:

MINERALS AND ELECTROLYTES

Discussion

 Minerals and electrolytes are essential for life and crucial for cellular function. They must be consumed on a regular basis in the diet for optimal health, but deficiencies in minerals and electrolytes are becoming part of the modern health dilemma.

Minerals are found in both food and water in varying amounts and chemical forms.

Minerals in the body are usually in the ionic, or electrically charged form, and are found in the fluids of the body and as components of organic and cellular matter, such as bone, phospholipids and red blood cells.

Minerals that occur in large amounts in the body are referred to as macrominerals. If they occur in much smaller amounts they are referred to as trace minerals or microminerals.

MACROMINERALS	MICRO OR TRACE MINERALS	
Calcium	Zinc	Chromium
Potassium	Iron	Copper
Sodium	Selenium	Molybdenum
Magnesium	Manganese	Boron

Electrolytes

Minerals can also be categorized in terms of how they behave in solution. An electrolyte is a mineral or molecule that develops an electrical charge when in a solution of water.

There are two main categories of electrolytes in the body, cations and anions. Cations carry a positive electrical charge in solution and anions carry a negative charge.

NOTES:

The following table lists the minerals and molecules that form these two groups:

CATIONS	ANIONS
Sodium (Na^{2+})	Chloride (Cl^-)
Potassium (K^+)	Bicarbonate (HCO_3^-)
Calcium (Ca^{2+})	Phosphate (HPO_4^-)
Magnesium (Mg^{2+})	Sulfate (SO_4^-)

Electrolytes are found both inside and outside the cell in varying quantities. For instance higher concentrations of potassium and magnesium are found inside the cell and higher concentrations of sodium and calcium are found outside the cell.

The movement of water with electrolytes across the cell membrane provides one of the main ways compounds move in and out of the cell. A good example of this is the sodium-potassium pump, which is the main electrolyte transport pump. It facilitates a myriad of essential functions, which includes fluid control, energy storage, acid/base balance, nerve conduction, muscle contraction and enzyme control.

Functions of Minerals

The body relies on a continuous supply of both macrominerals and trace minerals in order to function optimally. It is important to remember that the amount of minerals that are present in the body has no reflection on their relative importance. The following is a list of some of the functions of minerals:

1. Regulation of many enzymes by acting as co-factors

2. Maintaining acid/base balance

3. Maintaining osmotic pressure

4. Facilitating the transport of essential compounds across membranes

5. Maintaining nerve conduction

6. Maintaining muscle contraction

7. Regulation of tissue growth

8. Making up components of the body

9. Maintaining oxygen delivery and carbon dioxide excretion

NOTES:

Mineral Deficiency

Much of the information on the functions of minerals has come from the study of people who are deficient. Unfortunately mineral deficiency is becoming more and more common. The following is a list of some of the factors that cause mineral loss and mineral deficiency:

1. **Soil depletion-** the modern agri-chemical approach to farming has depleted our soils of many of the trace minerals.

2. **Modern food processing techniques-** Unfortunately enrichment of food does nothing to replace trace minerals lost during processing

3. **Digestive dysfunction-** digestive dysfunction is a very common clinical finding. If we lack the ability to breakdown our food properly we will not be able to separate the minerals from our food for absorption

4. **Mineral displacement from the body-** minerals are displaced from the body by many of the lifestyle choices we make e.g. coffee, sodas, sugar, alcohol displace key minerals. Chronic acid/base imbalances will also displace many minerals from the body.

5. **Drugs-** the birth control pill will antagonize zinc, diuretics can cause potassium loss

6. **Poor assimilation**

7. **Competition from heavy metals-** heavy metals, such as mercury, will prevent the uptake and storage of some minerals.

Tests for Mineral Deficiency

In the Functional Terrain Analysis there are a number of simple tests that can be used to determine if there are mineral deficiencies/insufficiencies, and if so, which minerals. The following is a list of these tests:

1. **Zinc Taste Test-** The zinc taste test can help identify zinc insufficiencies. Zinc insufficiency, if found, should be treated in all patients.

2. **Tissue Mineral Assessment Test-** a test for mineral insufficiency that helps to identify the correct forms of minerals the body needs, and if necessary what co-factors are needed.

3. **Dr. Kane's Mineral Assessment Tests-** a battery of screening tests that can help identify if any minerals are insufficient after a course of therapy has been completed. We recommend using this test after the other tests have been done.

NOTES:

ZINC TASTE TEST (ZTT, ZINC TALLY TEST)

The importance of zinc

Before we discuss this test, we would like to take a closer look at the importance of zinc in human nutrition.

Zinc is probably one of the most important trace minerals. Its effects on the body are far-reaching due to its role in more enzyme systems than the rest of all the trace minerals combined.

Zinc deficiency can lead to unnecessary suffering, which is why the zinc taste test is such an important method of assessing zinc deficiency in the body.

Zinc is a major component of over 70 metalloenzyme complexes, which catalyze major biochemical reactions in the body. One of the most important of these is carbonic anhydrase, the enzyme that catalyzes the carbonic acid-bicarbonate buffering system, without which we would not survive.

Zinc is also essential in the maintenance of our basal metabolic rate and zinc deficiency has been associated with a decreased Basal Metabolic Rate (BMR).

Despite its essentiality in life processes, no functional store of zinc appears to exist. Most of the body's zinc is locked away in bone and protein.

Key metabolic functions of zinc:

1. **Tissue growth** by regulation of protein synthesis

2. **Skin integrity and bone formation**

3. **Immune system-** Cell-mediated and generalized host defense

4. **Critical for cellular processes of replication, transcription and translation**

5. **Prevention of peroxide damage-** stabilization of membranes and fatty acids

6. **Night vision-** zinc is essential for the conversion of retinol into retinal

7. **Carbohydrate metabolism-** zinc deficiency causes a decreased insulin response and an impaired glucose tolerance

8. **Essential for delta-6-desaturase activity-** the enzyme that converts omega-3 and Omega-6 fatty acids

NOTES:

Zinc deficiency

Zinc deficiency is very common and becoming more widespread. Some of the reasons for zinc deficiency include:

- Birth control pills

- Impaired absorption- hypochlorhydria

- Alcoholism

- Kidney disease

- Increased dietary protein and phosphorous

- High intake of iron

- High phytate diets

- Steroid prescriptions

- Poor minerals in soil

Signs of zinc deficiency

Zinc deficiency has a large impact on the body and cellular function, owing to the importance that zinc plays in human metabolism. Some of the signs of zinc deficiency include:

1. Loss of taste and smell

2. Failure to thrive

3. Reduced immunity

4. Reproductive difficulties- decrease in sexual function of men

5. Loss of appetite

6. Skin disorders- seborrhea, scaling or flaking, acne

NOTES:

Zinc Taste Test- Discussion

 The Zinc Taste Test is a non-invasive method of determining a patient's physiological zinc status. It is a functional assessment as opposed to the quantitative assessment for zinc, such as serum or plasma zinc studies.

Zinc deficiency is strongly associated with a loss of taste acuity and this lack of "gustatory sensitivity" has been shown to be a possible indication of the "functional" availability of zinc.

A percentage of patients presenting with functional zinc deficiency are also deficient in vitamin B6 and magnesium, synergistic nutrients with zinc. If a patient fails the ZTT and does not respond to zinc therapy, they should be evaluated for B6 and magnesium status to find out the cause of the problem.

An initial short course of liquid zinc therapy is clinically more useful than tableted zinc, due to the fact that HCl production is also zinc dependent and tableted zinc may not be absorbed due to hypochlorhydria.

When to run this test?

1.   A non-invasive, quick and in-expensive method to assess a patient's zinc status

Source of Zinc Taste Test

1.   I recommend using the aqueous zinc product from Biotics Research.

2.   The Aqueous zinc is a zinc sulfate heptahydrate and in my experience is the best source for the Zinc Taste Test.

3.   Call Biotics at 1-800-231-5777 for the closest distributor.

Directions

1.   Patient's mouth should be free of any strong tastes

2.   Patient holds and swishes ¼ ounce of aqueous zinc in their mouth

3.   Start timing and have patient indicate when they first taste the solution

4.   Have them swallow after 15 seconds

5.   Ask them to describe the strength of taste or presence of an after taste

6.   Record strength of taste and seconds it took to taste the solution

NOTES:

Ranges

Level	Interpretation	Description
1	**Optimal Zinc levels**	**An immediate, unpleasant and obviously adverse taste in a few seconds (strongly metallic)**
2	**Mild zinc deficiency**	**A definite but not strongly unpleasant taste is noted in 4-6 seconds and tends to intensify with time. (delayed metallic)**
3	**Moderate Zinc Deficient**	**No taste noted initially, but develops in 7-13 seconds. May be described as sweet or bitter**
4	**Very Zinc Deficient**	**Tasteless or "tastes like water".**

Clinical implications

Levels 3 or 4 represent a zinc deficiency and should be treated by following the following zinc challenge protocol.

Zinc Challenge

- The zinc challenge is used to assess how zinc deficient your patient may be and how much zinc therapy is needed.

- The zinc challenge uses repeated challenges with the aqueous zinc to determine how much aqueous zinc is needed to begin supplementation.

- Aqueous zinc can be used therapeutically in the initial stages of zinc supplementation. Although low dose, it is an optimal form to enhance zinc absorption. It is much less dependent on optimal hydrochloric acid levels than other forms of zinc

Zinc Challenge Directions

- Begin with standard the Zinc Taste test as previously described

- Repeat the process successively, resting 30 seconds between tests, and noting changes in strength of taste

- Note how many challenges it takes for the patient to reach a strong metallic taste indicating zinc saturation

NOTES:

- We can approximate that the number of challenges will equal the number of bottles of aqueous zinc that the patient needs to begin a zinc maintenance program

- Dosage for aqueous zinc supplementation is 1 ounce 2X/day with meals

- After the course of aqueous zinc begin supplementation with 45 mg of zinc 2 times a day for 60 days. At this time redo the ZTT.

If patient is unable to reach a metallic taste with the zinc challenge consider the following options:

1. Treat presumptively if zinc deficiency signs are present

2. Screen with white blood cell zinc and magnesium levels (a synergistic nutrient with zinc)

3. Rule out Vitamin B6 deficiency with serum homocysteine

4. If indicated start treating with B6 and Magnesium

5. Consider damaged olfactory centers, which compromise the ability to taste and smell (trauma, smoking)

Zinc is best taken with meals to prevent nausea, which is most often seen in people who are both zinc deficient and hypochlorhydric

Interfering Factors

Vitamin B6 or Magnesium deficiency can cause a false positive result.

Related Tests

- Serum or plasma zinc studies

- Red or white blood cell zinc

- Homocysteine

- White or red blood cell magnesium

- Alkaline phosphatase on a chemistry screen

NOTES:

TISSUE MINERAL ASSESSMENT TEST

Background

The Tissue Mineral Assessment test provides a way to check tissue mineral stores in individuals suspected of having a tissue mineral insufficiency. The test uses the presence of muscle cramping as a sign of low tissue calcium levels. Muscle tetany is an indication of tissue mineral insufficiency in the muscle spindle fibers. If a deficiency is confirmed, various forms of calcium and other minerals and co-factors are tested orally using a biofeedback test called Neuro-Lingual Testing in order to determine which specific forms of minerals and nutrients are needed to improve tissue mineral status.

Mineral status depends on more than just getting the right mineral. Other factors such as digestion, absorption and assimilation are essential too. Testing co-factors such as stomach hydrochloric acid, essential fatty acids, vitamins or hormonal remedies can improve the mineral status.

The Tissue Mineral Assessment test is ultimately screening for multiple factors in calcium metabolism at the tissue level. Serum calcium levels are too tightly regulated to be of clinical use in measuring tissue calcium status.

Discussion

Calcium is essential for bone metabolism, the drawing of fats through the intestinal wall and protein absorption. Calcium is mobilized by the body in trauma, infections, and stress, and is used rapidly for repair of tissue in conjunction with vitamin A, vitamin C, magnesium, phosphorus, iodine and unsaturated fatty acids.

- Calcium is one of the alkaline minerals and is used as a buffer by the body.

- Calcium increases sympathetic output by stimulating the sympathetic nervous system.

- Optimal levels of calcium are needed to support the skeletal, muscular, and nervous system.

- An imbalance in calcium can create anxiety, nervousness, irritability, insomnia, muscle tension, spasms or cramps, low back pain, constipation, and hypertension or heart palpitations.

- Many people will test low in calcium, including those who eat organic whole foods and take calcium supplements.

NOTES:

- There is a predominant belief that calcium deficiency is very common and that most patients would benefit from daily supplementation. Clinical experience suggests that a calcium need has less to do with calcium deficiency and more to do with an inability to absorb and utilize dietary calcium.

- Rule out hypochlorhydria, the need for magnesium, phosphorous, vitamin A, B and C, unsaturated fatty acids, and iodine as some of the reasons for a "calcium" need, before supplementing with calcium.

- When subjective indicators or lab testing identify a potential calcium need, the lack of synergistic co-factors that aid in calcium metabolism is often the main problem.

Common subjective indications of calcium need are:

- Muscle cramps at rest

- Frequent nose bleeds

- Soft fingernails

- Frequent cold sores, skin rashes, sunburn or hives

- High or low blood pressure.

- Irritability

- Fever with a mild cold or virus

- Frequent hoarseness

Calcium Regulation- a need for co-factors

Calcium regulation in the body is determined by a number of different co-factors that are necessary for adequate digestion, absorption, and utilization of calcium. These include:

1. Digestion

Calcium and other minerals require Hydrochloric Acid (HCl) for uptake. Ensuring adequate stomach function can increase calcium absorption from the diet.

2. Vitamin D

Vitamin D acts to increase calcium levels in the blood by increasing calcium uptake from the gut, by pulling calcium from the tissue and decreasing fecal and urinary calcium loss

NOTES:

3. Essential Fatty Acid

Essential fatty acids help increase tissue calcium levels and are necessary for the transport of calcium across the cell membrane into the cells

4. Systemic pH

Calcium is a major buffer of blood pH and as such is affected by changes in blood pH.

When the blood becomes too alkaline, calcium precipitates out of solution and can be deposited in excess into inappropriate tissue:

- **Eyes**—cataracts

- **Bones**—bone spurs

- **Joints**—bursitis

- **Kidneys**—stones

When the blood becomes too acidic, calcium is resorbed from tissue, which can cause problems in the following areas:

- **Skin**—cold sores, herpes, sunburn, canker sores, etc.

- **Teeth**—dental caries, gum problems

- **Bones**—osteoporosis

5. Calcium must be in balance with the other macro minerals

Phosphorous is the opposing acid mineral

Magnesium is often deficient in the American diet, and is important for the body to appropriately use calcium

6. Trace minerals are also important in the utilization of Calcium:

Manganese, boron, copper, zinc, potassium

7. Hormones

Calcium metabolism is affected and regulated by a number of different hormones

Parathyroid hormone (PTH)

NOTES:

- PTH increases serum Calcium levels by increasing calcium uptake from the gut, by pulling calcium from tissue, by decreasing urinary and fecal loss of calcium and by increasing osteoclastic activity in the bone.

Calcitonin

- Calcitonin is secreted from the thyroid gland and has a weak effect of blood calcium. It inhibits osteolytic activity of the osteoclasts and promotes calcium deposition in the bone, thereby decreasing blood calcium levels+

Sex hormones

- The sex hormones' effect on calcium metabolism is due to their effect on bone metabolism

- Progesterone and estrogen promote bone building and therefore may lead to a decrease in serum calcium.

- Testosterone promotes calcium retention in the bone and may cause a decrease in serum calcium.

When would you run this test?

- To check tissue calcium and mineral need

- To test which mineral or co-factor is needed to correct mineral insufficiency.

Directions

- Place a standard blood pressure cuff around the patient's calf muscle

- Instruct the patient to let you know when the feel the ONSET of cramping pain.

- Gradually inflate the cuff

- Stop and deflate immediately when the threshold is reached

- Record the number and wait 30 seconds and repeat the test to verify the baseline

- Have patient perform a neuro-lingual test on a chosen mineral or co-factor supplement and then re-check Lowenburg's test to see if there is improvement

- The correct mineral and co-factor, if necessary, will bring the Lowenburg's test within the optimal range of 220-240 mmHg

NOTES:

NOTE: Do not use this test if peripheral vascular disease is suspected or present. In elderly or frail patients do not exceed 180 mmHg

Results

< 200 mmHg: patient is deficient

200-220 mmHg: Patient is sufficient

220-240: Optimal

It is not necessary to test the cramping threshold beyond 240

Clinical implications

< 220mmHg

Clinical Implication	Additional information
Patient is deficient or just sufficient in a mineral or co-factor	If a deficiency is confirmed, various forms of calcium and other minerals and co-factors can be tested orally using a biofeedback test called Neuro-Lingual Testing in order to determine which specific forms of minerals and nutrients are needed to improve tissue mineral status. Use the Neuro-Lingual Test (NLT) to challenge the Tissue Mineral Assessment test with various different supplements and co-factors until the number is brought up into the optimal range of 220-240 mmHg.

Interfering Factors

Vascular insufficiency in lower extremities may interfere with test.

Related Tests

- Zinc Taste Test

- Dr. Bieler's Salivary pH Acid Challenge

NOTES:

NEURO-LINGUAL TESTING

Background

There is a powerful connection between the sensory organs and the Central Nervous System (CNS). Sensory organ innervation represents some of the most evolved and highly specialized systems in the body. Stimulation of the sensory organs e.g. sight, smell, touch etc. has a wide range of effects on human physiology. Sensory innervation is primarily located in the limbic system, the survival center of the brain. Our primary means of interacting with our environment are made via these sensory innervations. One of the most highly innervated sensory systems is the sense of taste.

Taste discrimination is essential for survival as this is often the first means of the brain to interpret value or harm. Experiments have shown that adrenalectomized animals automatically select water with a high concentration of sodium chloride, animals injected with insulin select the sweetest foods among many samples, and parathyroidectomized animals automatically select water with a high concentration of calcium chloride. There are also strong neuro-limbic memories created by harmful substances i.e. poisons, spoiled foods etc.

These experiments underscore the brain's ability to determine physiological need via sensory pathways i.e. taste discrimination. Some nutritional supplements are essentially food concentrates, which can be introduced as a stimulus to the CNS via the lingual pathways (Neuro-Lingual Testing or NLT).

Discussion

 On first application of a taste stimulus a nerve impulse is generated within a fraction of a second.

The nerve impulse travels via the lingual and/or glossopharyngeal nerves to the Tractus Solarius in the brain stem, which generates multiple impulses that travel into the brain stem.

The brain in turn sends many efferent messages to multiple control mechanisms throughout the body.

The CNS communicates with many tissues and organs within the body to regulate or restore function.

The Tissue Mineral Assessment test responds well to the Neuro-Lingual testing of the correct combination of minerals and co-factors.

NOTES:

With the right combination of minerals and co-factors the muscle cramping threshold will increase. It is important to remember that a positive response to the NLT does not occur through absorption of the nutrient; rather change occurs via the neurological connection between the CNS, the lingual pathways, and the peripheral system.

NOTES:

DR. KANE'S MINERAL ASSESSMENT TESTS

Discussion

 Dr. Kane's mineral assessment tests can be used as a follow-up to the Zinc Taste Test and Tissue Mineral Assessment test. We recommend using it to track down and treat minerals that may still remain deficient after being on a mineral replacement program. We use this test after a few months of having a patient on a mineral replacement program.

The test is based on the principle that our taste has intelligence. We know from the success of the Neuro-Lingual Testing how powerful this phenomenon is. These tests use the sense of taste as a guide. The cells in the mouth act as ionic probes and are exquisitely sensitive. They record and send back signals to the Central nervous system (CNS) on the different chemical contents of foods we take in. Dr. Kane used this concept in developing the mineral assessment tests and developed a group of essential minerals in the correct concentrations to enable us to use this feedback system to determine mineral need.

The test kits allow you to test for the following minerals:

1. **Potassium**
2. **Zinc**
3. **Magnesium**
4. **Copper**

5. **Chromium**
6. **Manganese**
7. **Molybdenum**
8. **Selenium**

When would you run this test?

- As a follow-up to test for mineral insufficiency

Directions

- Start with bottle #1, pour a small amount in a glass or cup, and hold in the mouth

- The patient notes their response to the mineral test using the following scale:

	Taste Test Score	Clinical implication
1	Sweet	Definitely need the mineral
2	Pleasant	Need the mineral
3	No Taste	Need the mineral
4	Hmmmm…taste something	Sufficient
5	So-So, there is some taste	Do not need mineral
6	Don't like	Do not need mineral
7	Gross taste	Do not need mineral

NOTES:

- Write down the appropriate response on the score card

- Repeat this process for each of the remaining minerals

Functions of the minerals included in the test kit:

Potassium

1. Acid/base balance

2. Electrical activity of nerve and muscle cell function

3. Water balance

4. Movement of nutrients across cell membrane

5. Kidney and adrenal function

6. Heart function

7. Converting blood sugar into glycogen

8. Regulation of blood pressure

Zinc

1. Regulates liver release of vitamin A

2. Involved in DNA and RNA synthesis

3. Essential for cell growth

4. Prostate health requires zinc

5. Vision

6. Multiple enzymatic co-factors

7. Immune function

8. Crucial for taste perception

9. Protects against heavy metal toxicity e.g. cadmium and mercury

Copper

1. Acts as a co-factor in various enzymatic reactions

NOTES:

2. Essential for collagen cross linking and connective tissue repair

3. Breakdown of Estrogenic hormones

4. Neurotransmitter production

5. Melanin production

6. An important component of the free radical scavenger SOD

Chromium

1. Essential component of Glucose Tolerance Factor, which helps potentiate insulin function

Manganese

1. Needed for muscle and bone function

2. Skin integrity

3. Bone remodeling

4. Pancreatic and brain function

5. Protection of oxidative damage in mitochondria

6. Carbohydrate and lipid metabolism

Magnesium

1. Regulation of calcium absorption

2. Structural integrity of bones and teeth

3. Regulation of contractility of heart muscle

4. Muscle relaxation

5. Decreases blood coagulation

6. Acts as a calcium channel blocker

7. Co-factor in essential fatty acid metabolism

8. Enhances immune function

9. Involved in energy metabolism (ATP)

NOTES:

Molybdenum

1.   A co-factor in redox reactions

2.   A co-factor in the following enzymes:

3.   Sulfite oxidase- essential for conversion of sulfites into sulfates and metabolism of sulfur containing amino acids

4.   Xanthine oxidase- detoxification and production of uric acid as the enzyme responsible for terminal oxidation of purines

5.   Aldehyde oxidase- enzyme responsible for detoxifying alcohol

Selenium

1.   Essential for the production of glutathione peroxidase

2.   Has been shown to inhibit certain types of cancer

3.   Immuno-stimulating: stimulates production of antibodies

4.   Necessary for sexual function

5.   Protection from toxic effects of heavy metals

Clinical uses of selenium:

- o   Prevention of cancer

- o   Arthritis

- o   Allergy desensitization

- o   Detoxification

- o   Cardiovascular disease

- o   Heavy metal toxicity

- o   Eye disorders: cataracts, macular degeneration

- o   Prevention of viral illness

NOTES:

Results

Normal/sufficient: A mild to strong taste

Insufficient: Little to no taste, or a sweet /pleasant taste

Clinical implications

Clinical Implication	Additional information
Specific mineral insufficiency	The results should be viewed in conjunction with the other mineral assessment tests and relevant co-factors to mineral use should be considered. However, supplementation in a strongly deficient result should prove useful.

Related Tests

- Zinc Taste Test
- Tissue Mineral Test
- Whole Blood Mineral Assessment

Adrenal
Terrain

NOTES:

ADRENAL TERRAIN AND THE STRESS RESPONSE

Background

The adrenal system evolved to deal with acute and/or emergency situations of "fight or flight". It was never intended to be the primary response to stress. Adrenal problems are very prevalent in modern society, particularly functional adrenal problems. Western medicine looks at the adrenals in terms of pathological extremes. Your adrenals are either healthy or you have one of two problems: Cushing's syndrome (a disease of an extreme excess cortisol output) or Addison's disease (a disease of deficient cortisol output). Adrenal dysfunction is rarely primary, but rather secondary to metabolic dysfunction elsewhere.

Physiology

- The adrenal glands are two small endocrine organs that lie on top of the kidneys.

- The gland is composed of two distinct areas, the cortex in the outer layer and the medulla in the inner layer.

- Each layer is responsible for producing various types of hormones.

- The cortex produces corticosteroid hormones, which include the mineralcorticoids (aldosterone), Glucocorticoids (cortisol), and anabolic and sex hormones (DHEA).

- The medulla produces catecholamines (Epinephrine and Norepinephrine).

NOTES:

The Main Adrenal Hormones

The three main hormones we will be talking about are Cortisol, DHEA and Aldosterone.

Cortisol

- Cortisol activity is regulated by the hypothalamic-pituitary-adrenal axis.

- Secretion of cortisol is stimulated by the release of Adrenocorticotropic hormone (ACTH) from the pituitary.

- ACTH is regulated by Corticotropin releasing factor (CRF) released by the hypothalamus. A feedback inhibition loop exists between CRF and ACTH.

- Cortisol levels fluctuate over the day and night according to the circadian rhythms, which are regulated by the sleep-wake cycle. A steep increase in cortisol output occurs in the morning, peaking at approximately 8 a.m. This is followed by a tapering off until midnight, when cortisol levels are at their lowest.

Functions of cortisol include:

1. Mobilizes and increases amino acids in blood and liver by promoting protein catabolism

2. Stimulates liver to convert amino acids to glucose

3. Stimulates increased glycogen in the liver

4. Inhibits glucose utilization in the peripheral tissue

5. Mobilizes and increases fatty acids in the blood by supporting synthesis of hormone sensitive lipase

6. Counters inflammation and allergies

7. Prevents loss of sodium in urine and helps maintain blood volume and blood pressure

8. Sustains tissue responsiveness to catecholamines

9. Maintains resistance to stress

10. Maintains personality and emotional stability

11. Modulates thyroid function

NOTES:

DHEA

- Dehydroepiandrosterone (DHEA) is primarily produced from the adrenal cortex.

- It is produced from the steroid precursor pregnenolone, which is synthesized from cholesterol.

- DHEA has a very short half life (about 30 minutes) and subsequently about 95% of circulating DHEA is in the more stable sulfate form DHEA-S.

- DHEA-S follows a similar daily circadian rhythm to cortisol, but it shows a less well defined pattern over the course of the month.

- DHEA-S levels may respond to seasonal changes. Higher levels of DHEA-S have been recorded from autumn to spring.

Functions of DHEA include:

1. Acting as an androgen with anabolic activity

2. Precursor to testosterone

3. Precursor to estrogen and progesterone

4. Reverses immune suppression caused by excessive cortisol level and therefore improves resistance to viruses, bacteria, candida albicans, parasites, allergies and cancer

5. Stimulates bone deposition and remodeling, which can help prevent osteoporosis

6. Improves cardiovascular status by lowering total and LDL cholesterol levels, lessens incidence of heart attack

7. Increases muscle mass

8. Decreases percentage body fat

9. Reverses many of the unfavorable effects of excess cortisol

10. Can help create an improvement in: energy, vitality, sleep, PMS, and mental clarity

11. Can help with quicker recovery from any kind of acute stress: insufficient sleep, excessive exercise, mental strain etc.

NOTES:

Aldosterone

- Aldosterone is produced in the Zona glomerulosa in the adrenal cortex and is the most important mineralocorticoid hormone.

- Mineralcorticoids regulate the transport of sodium (Na^+) and potassium (K^+) in the kidney and other organs (gall bladder, intestines, sweat glands, salivary glands etc.).

- The levels of aldosterone in the body fluctuate according to Sodium chloride (NaCl) intake and the time of the day.

- The rate of its secretion is at its highest in the early morning and is lowest in the late evening, a pattern that is not dissimilar to cortisol.

- The release of aldosterone is stimulated by a reduction in blood volume, hyponatremia (low sodium in the blood), hyperkalemia (high potassium in the blood) and the action of Angiotensin II.

- ACTH also stimulates the formation of aldosterone.

Functions of aldosterone include:

1. Increases sodium retention throughout the body

2. Increases potassium excretion

3. Increases water retention

4. Increases extracellular volume

5. Enhances the activity of the sodium/potassium pump

6. Helps "bring on line" the sodium and potassium channels in the luminal membrane in the kidneys

Adrenal dysfunction and the stress response

- The adrenal hormones not only play an enormous and pivotal role in the body's ability to respond and adapt to stress but their own production becomes severely impacted by long term stress.

- Chronic and/or severe stress causes an individual to undergo the "general adaptation syndrome" first proposed by Dr. Hans Selye. If the stress is not relieved they may well end up suffering from adrenal hypofunction or adrenal insufficiency.

NOTES:

What are some of the adrenal stressors?

External Stressors	Internal or Physiological	Mental
• Toxic exposure • Light cycle disruptions • Allergies • Temperature extremes • Trauma • Overwork (physical and/or mental)	• Dietary imbalances: increased refined carbohydrates • Nutrient deficiencies • Lack of sleep • Blood sugar dysregulation • Chronic infections • Pain • Excessive exercise • Chronic inflammation	• Emotional strain: anger, fear, worry, guilt • Anxiety • Depression •

NOTES:

The Stages of the Stress Response

The stress response progresses through a number of different adaptive stages before fatigue sets in. The stress response can be divided into three stages:

1. The alarm reaction

2. The Compensation/decompensation stage (Adrenal hyperfunction)

3. The Fatigue Stage (adrenal hypofunction)

The Alarm Reaction

The alarm reaction is the normal stress response and has the following characteristics:

*   The sympathetic nervous system responds to stressors within seconds, causing the release of catecholamines (Epinephrine and Norepinephrine) from the adrenal medulla, which get the body into a "fight or flight" mode.

*   The catecholamines stimulate the hypothalamic-pituitary system causing the release of ACTH

*   ACTH stimulates the adrenal cortex causing the release of cortisol and increases the levels of free cortisol in the body

*   ACTH also causes an increase in DHEA from the adrenal cortex

*   Increased cortisol acts on the pituitary to stop the further release of ACTH and thereby quietening the stress response

*   The cortisol and the catecholamines cause short-tem high blood sugar via the action on the liver to breakdown glycogen increase gluconeogenesis and breakdown fat.

*   The increased steroid hormones return to normal after the stressor is removed

NOTES:

THE NORMAL STRESS RESPONSE

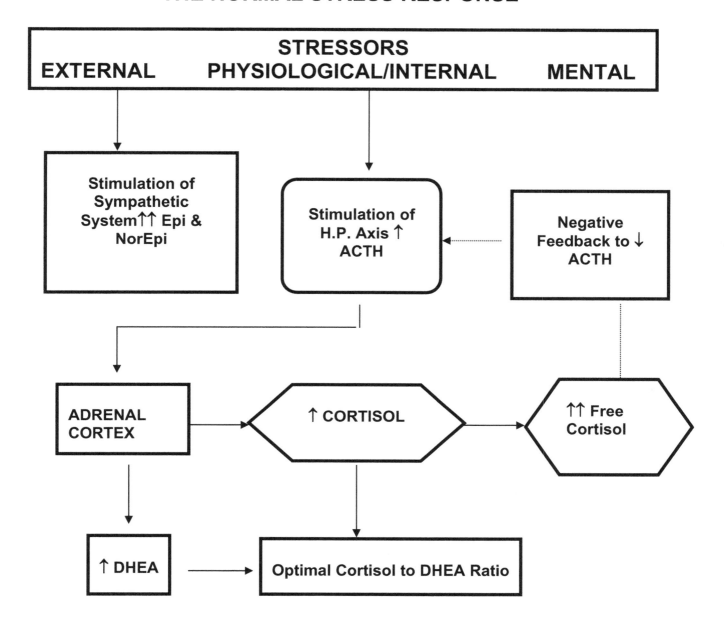

NOTES:

The Compensation stage moving towards decompensation (Adrenal hyper-function)

The compensation phase sets in when the above stressors are not removed and the cortisol levels remain high in relation to the DHEA levels. This stage has the following characteristics:

- The sympathetic nervous system still responds to the stressors and continues to cause the release of catecholamines (Epinephrine and Norepinephrine) from the adrenal medulla.

- The catecholamines stimulate the hypothalamic-pituitary system causing the continued release of ACTH

- ACTH stimulates the adrenal cortex causing the release of cortisol and increases the levels of free cortisol in the body

- The hypothalamic-pituitary system normally responds to increased cortisol levels by decreasing ACTH output. In the compensation stage hypothalamus-pituitary system begins to get insensitive to the presence of cortisol and cortisol levels continue to stay high.

- DHEA levels, instead of rising like the cortisol, remain normal or show no signs of increase leading to an increased cortisol/DHEA ratio that is out of balance.

- cortisol leads to adrenal hyperfunctioning

- Decompensation begins to occur as the levels of DHEA begin to decrease due the failure of the adrenal cortex to produce DHEA upon ACTH stimulation

NOTES:

COMPENSATION/DECOMPENSATION PHASE OR ELEVATED CORTISOL TO DHEA RATIO

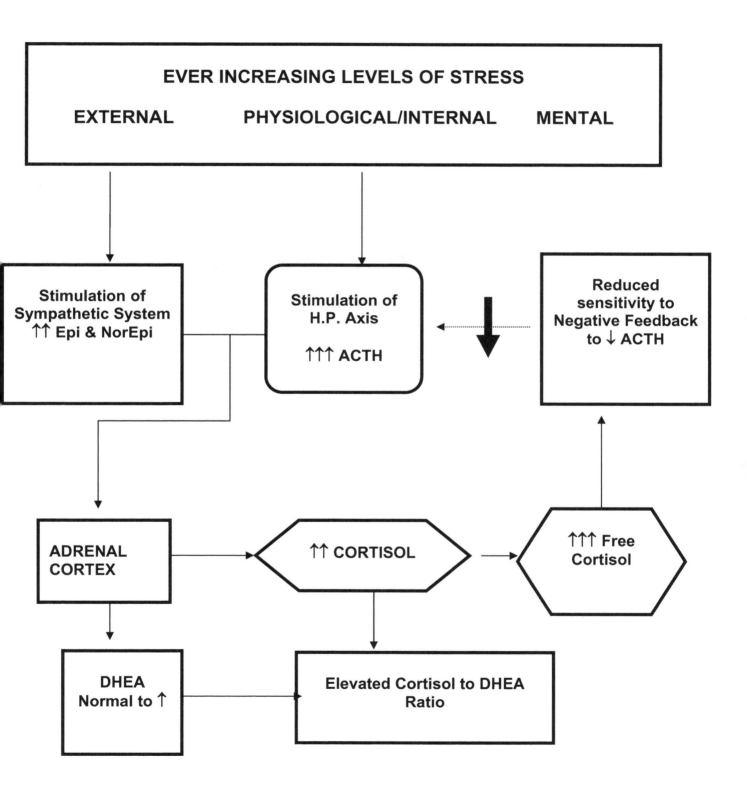

NOTES:

Signs and symptoms of Adrenal Hyperfunction

1. Decreased insulin sensitivity leading to increased insulin resistance

2. Diminished glucose utilization by cell

3. Increased blood sugar levels

4. Salt and water retention due to excess aldosterone activity

5. Decreased protein synthesis

6. Increased gluconeogenesis: increased protein and fat breakdown leading to muscle wasting

7. Increased bone loss (osteoporosis)

8. Increased infections: chronic EBV, CMV

9. Shrinking of lymphatic tissue

10. Diminished lymphocyte numbers and functions

11. Decreased secretory antibody production (Secretory IgA)

12. Decreased immune function, which can lead to allergies, infections and cancer

13. Weight gain around the abdomen due to fat and water retention

14. Increased LDL cholesterol levels

15. Muscle wasting

16. Allergies

17. Insomnia

18. Reduced vitality

19. Hunger

20. PMS and other hormonal problems

NOTES:

The Fatigue Stage (adrenal hypofunction)

The fatigue stage sets in when the stressors continue to act on the body, which can no longer react, causing decreased cortisol and DHEA output. This stage has the following characteristics:

- The sympathetic nervous system continues to respond to the stressors and continues to cause the release of catecholamines (Epinephrine and Norepinephrine) from the adrenal medulla.

- The catecholamines continue to stimulate the hypothalamic-pituitary system causing the continued release of ACTH

- In the fatigue stage the hypothalamus-pituitary system is barely sensitive to the presence of cortisol.

- ACTH levels continue to stay high and continue to stimulate the adrenal glands. The adrenal cortex, at this stage, is so fatigued that it can no longer respond to ACTH stimulation, causing a dramatic decrease in the secretion of hormones.

- Free cortisol is decreased and DHEA is normal or decreased, which leads to a decreased cortisol/DHEA ratio

NOTES:

ADRENAL HYPOFUNCTION AND DECREASED CORTISOL TO DHEA RATIO

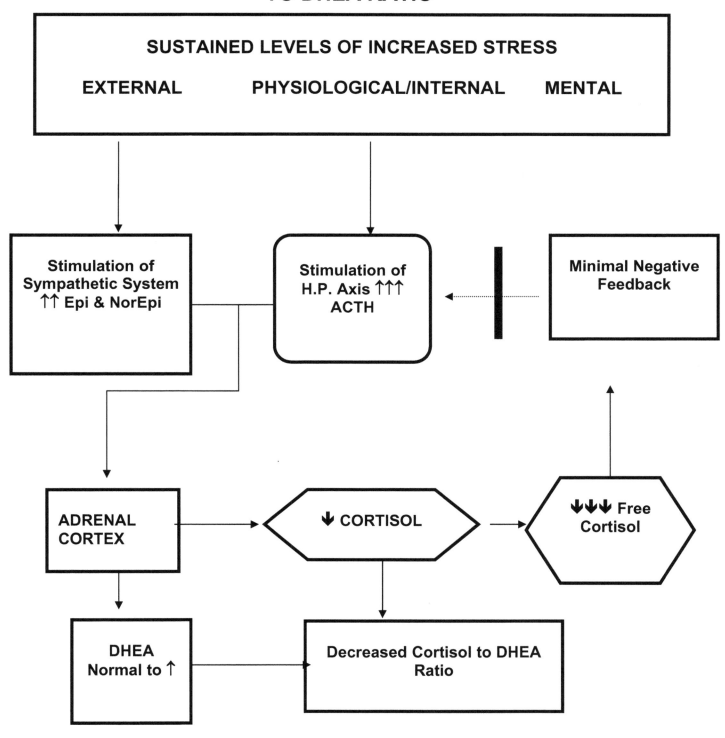

NOTES:

Signs and Symptoms Adrenal Hypofunction and of a decreased Cortisol/DHEA ratio

A decreased cortisol/DHEA ratio and adrenal hypofunctioning causes a decrease in gluconeogenesis, leading to hypoglycemia, hunger, depression, low energy and the following signs and symptoms:

1. Irritability

2. Allergies

3. Inflammation

4. Reactive hypoglycemia

5. Increased carbohydrate sensitivity

6. Low blood pressure

7. Chronic inflammation due to up regulation of pro-inflammatory mediators

8. Fatigue

9. Excessive anxiety and apprehension

10. Reduced ability to concentrate

11. Poor memory

12. PMS and menstrual irregularities

13. Alcohol intolerance

14. Heart palpitations

15. Digestive complaints e.g. dyspepsia

16. Increased oxidative stress and increased tissue damage

17. Degenerative diseases

NOTES:

Assessing for adrenal function

Adrenal function can be assessed in the office using the Urine Adrenal Stress Test or Koenisburg test for urinary chloride. Although it will not give specific information on cortisol and DHEA levels, it is a useful "gateway" test for the adrenal system. It is a valuable screening test before embarking on the more expensive salivary adrenal stress profiles offered by many of the alternative diagnostic laboratories. Use of Ragland's test for postural hypotension and the Paradoxical Pupillary Reflex test can give indications of long term adrenal balance.

1. Urinary Adrenal Stress Test

2. Ragland's Test for Postural Hypotension

3. Paradoxical Pupillary Reflex Test

NOTES:

URINARY ADRENAL STRESS TEST (Koenisburg test, Urinary chloride test)

Discussion

 The Urinary adrenal stress test measures the amount of chloride displaced into the urine. Increased or decreased levels of chloride in the urine are a useful way of assessing for adrenal stress or fatigue, kidney stress, mineral loss from the body and acid-alkaline imbalance.

Adrenal stress is a major health problem. Adrenal hyperfunctioning, as seen in the compensation stage of stress adaptation, leads to an increased output of adrenal hormones such as cortisol and aldosterone. High levels of aldosterone cause the resorption of sodium and chloride leading to low levels of sodium and chloride in the urine.

Adrenal hypofunctioning or fatigue, on the other hand, leads to a decreased output of cortisol and aldosterone. Low levels of aldosterone cause the increased loss of sodium and chloride into the urine. Exhausted adrenal glands can lead to chronic fatigue, chronic inflammations, a weakened immune system, problems with PMS, difficulties with blood pressure, be a contributing factor to insomnia and allergies as well as reducing the sex drive. The earlier the adrenal imbalances are cleared up, the more rapidly the patient's energy levels return to normal.

Poor sodium resorption causes an increased level of stress to the kidneys leading to possible kidney dysfunction.

The loss of sodium and chloride from the body follows the loss of magnesium and potassium i.e. if we already have a decreased urinary chloride, then we can presume that we have a decreased level of magnesium and potassium in the blood. The loss of these and other minerals leads to a loss of vital co-enzymes, essential for energy production in the cell.

When would you run this test?

1. To check a patients adrenal status

2. To get an idea of the energy output of the patient

3. To assess for kidney burden

4. To assess for mineral loss, especially potassium and magnesium

NOTES:

Directions

It is best to use the first morning urine. If patient is coming in later for an appointment, refrigerate in an airtight container. Patients should restrict salt intake for 2 days prior to testing.

1. Put 10 drops of urine into a small glass vial.

2. Add 1 drop of 20% Potassium Chromate—shake to mix.

3. Add 2.9% Silver Nitrate, one drop at a time—shake to mix.

4. Record the number of drops it takes to produce a deep brick red color i.e. no yellow color remaining.

Description of the test

This test determines the chloride ion concentration of the urine using a simple titration with silver nitrate. 10 drops of urine are used with 1 drop of potassium chromate. As the silver nitrate solution is added to the urine/potassium chromate a precipitate of silver chloride forms. The test becomes significant when the end point of the titration has been reached and the solution turns brick-red in color. At this point all of the chloride ions are precipitated and any additional silver ions react with the chromate to form a red-brown precipitate of silver chromate.

NOTE: This test is most accurate with a urine sample pH 6.5 and higher. If the urine pH is lower than pH 6.5 the chromate ions may be removed by an acid-base reaction to form hydrogen chromate ions or dichromate ions, affecting the accuracy of the test. **Please test the urine pH prior to doing this test and be aware that a low urine pH may make this test less accurate.**

Results

# of drops to produce color change	Interpretation
1 – 6 drops	Low urinary chloride
7 – 8 drops	Normal
> 8 drops	High urinary chloride

PLEASE NOTE: The reagents used in this test are the ones obtained from Rocky Mountain Reagents. Other companies may provide reagents for the Urine Chloride test but they use a different concentration of potassium chromate and silver nitrate so the

NOTES:

number of drops needed to get a change may be different. Please refer to their results chart and then use the clinical interpretations below.

Clinical implications

HIGH URINE CHLORIDE

Clinical Implication	Additional information
Adrenal hypofunctioning	Adrenal hypofunctioning causes a decrease in aldosterone secretion from the adrenal cortex, which leads to decreased sodium and chloride resorption, leading to an increased urine chloride.
Hypochlorhydria	The chloride should mainly be in the stomach as part of the HCL molecule. High urinary chloride may indicate a lack of chloride to be available for HCL production.
Kidney stress	Poor sodium and chloride resorption leads to an increased stress to the kidneys, contributing to kidney dysfunction.
Alkaline Mineral insufficiency	Increased loss of magnesium and other minerals in the urine precedes the loss of sodium and chloride from the body.
Oxidative stress	Adrenal hypofunctioning is associated with an increased level of oxidative stress in the body. Acute stress with no adrenal response will cause an increase in oxidative stress.
Conditions are associated with increased chloride	• Dehydration • Fasting and starvation • Diuretic use

NOTES:

LOW URINE CHLORIDE

Clinical Implication	Additional information
Adrenal hyperfunction	Excess aldosterone is secreted from the adrenal cortex in adrenal hyperfunctioning, leading to increased resorption of sodium and chloride, causing a decrease in urine chloride.
Electrolyte stress/ Increased toxicity	Excess aldosterone causes a decreased excretion of minerals, which can contribute to electrolyte/mineral stress and excess toxicity in the body
The following conditions are associated with decreased chloride	• Malabsorption syndrome • Pyloric obstruction • Diarrhea and /or vomiting and diaphoresis • Emphysema • Congestive heart failure

NOTES:

Interfering Factors

Levels vary with salt intake

Related Tests

- Please check Dr. Bieler's salivary pH acid challenge if high levels of stress are suspected.

- Check multi-stix if the test is greater than 8 drops. Please see my e-book *"Quick Reference Guide to Urine Dipstick Analysis and Functional Urinalysis"* for more details.

- Please check the Oxidata test for oxidative stress levels when Urine Chloride levels are low.

- Urine chloride can be used in conjunction with other tests. Please see the section of patterns for a more detailed description of patterns seen with Urine chloride.

NOTES:

RAGLAND'S POSTURAL HYPOTENSION TEST

Discussion

 Ragland's test for postural hypotension is used to determine the presence and severity of adrenal exhaustion or hypoadrenia.

It assesses the body's ability to compensate for the hydrostatic effects of gravity by measuring a drop in systolic blood pressure from a recumbent to a standing position.

Standing from a recumbent position causes pressure changes in the vascular system, which are controlled by the splanchnic veins.

The splanchnic veins, being devoid of valves, are dependent upon nerve function, for their tone.

The tone of the splanchnic nerves is under the direct control of the adrenal system.

When would you run this test?

- To check a patients adrenal status

Directions

1. Instruct the patient to lay supine on the treatment table

2. Place the blood pressure cuff on the arm of choice, determine the systolic pressure and release the pressure

3. Pump up the cuff again 15 mmHg higher than the supine systolic pressure and while supporting their arm, instruct the patient to stand up quickly

4. Immediately release the valve so that you can determine the standing systolic pressure within 5 seconds of the patient arising.

5. The test may be conducted sitting to standing but the BP may not drop as dramatically. Results may be halved.

6. You may want to repeat the standing BP after one minute to see how they are compensating.

NOTES:

Results

Result	Clinical Implication
Excellent	**Result:** 6-10 point increase in systolic blood pressure upon standing **Implication:** An optimal response- good adrenal health. Consider that this may actually be the beginning of the alarm stage of adrenal exhaustion. The patient is compensating ok but in early stages of decompensation. If this continues you may see a BP drop.
Fair	**Result:** Systolic pressure remains the same **Implication:** Fair adrenal compensation
Poor	**Result:** Systolic pressure drops up to 10 points **Implication:** Beginning to see long term adrenal dysfunction
Failure	**Result:** Systolic pressure drops up to 20 points **Implication:** Adrenal fatigue
Exhaustion	**Result:** Systolic pressure drops over 20 points **Implication:** Adrenal fatigue probably very pronounced. **NOTE:** Repeat standing BP after one minute to see if there is additional compensation to bring BP under control. Some will decrease further, which is a problem

NOTES:

Clinical implications

Clinical Implication	Additional information
Adrenal hypofunction	The autonomic nervous system control of pressure changes in the vascular system becomes compromised as adrenal output is diminished in adrenal hypofunction and exhaustion

Interfering Factors

1. Neuropathic hypotension from neurological and other diseases (e.g. DM) can cause orthostatic hypotension

2. Decreased blood volume and anemia

3. Drugs and diseases that interfere with the autonomic regulation of vascular pressure changes

Related Tests

- Urine adrenal stress test (urine chloride)

- Paradoxical Pupillary Response Test

- Adrenal Stress Index test (salivary measurement of cortisol and DHEA levels over a 24 hour period)

NOTES:

PARADOXICAL PUPILLARY RESPONSE TEST

Discussion

The paradoxical pupillary response test is used to determine the presence and severity of adrenal exhaustion.

The test is used to determine the presence and severity of adrenal exhaustion. It measures the ability of the pupil of the eye to respond to light.

A reduced ability of the pupil to constrict with light stimulus is a reflection of the "tug of war" between the sympathetic and parasympathetic branches of the autonomic nervous system

Pupillary constriction is strongly influenced by the hormonal cascade from the adrenal system

When would you run this test?

- To check a patients adrenal status

Directions

1. Darken the room and wait 15 seconds

2. Instruct the patient to look at a fixed point and not to blink

3. Come in from the side of the eye and direct the pen light at the pupil at approximately a 45° angle. Hold the light 6-12 inches from the patient's eye depending on the intensity of the light

4. Observe the reaction of the pupil for 20 seconds

NOTES:

Results

Result	Description	Implication
Excellent	Pupil constricts and holds tight for 20 seconds without pulsing	An optimal response- good adrenal health
Fair	Pupil holds but pulses after 10 seconds	Fair adrenal compensation
Poor	Pupil pulses and becomes larger after 5-10 seconds	Beginning to see long term adrenal dysfunction
Failure	Pupil pulses and becomes gradually larger over the first 10 seconds	Adrenal fatigue
Exhaustion	Pupil immediately becomes larger or fails to constrict	Adrenal fatigue probably very pronounced

Clinical implications

Clinical Implication	Additional information
Adrenal hypofunction and exhaustion	The autonomic nervous system control of the pupil's ability to react to light becomes compromised as adrenal output is diminished in adrenal hypofunction and exhaustion

Interfering Factors

1. Drugs and neurological dysfunction can interfere with the autonomic regulation of pupillary constriction in response to light

Related Tests

- Urine adrenal stress test (urine chloride),

- Ragland's Postural Hypotension Test,

- Adrenal Stress Index test (salivary measurement of cortisol and DHEA levels over a 24 hour period)

Thyroid
Terrain

NOTES:

THYROID TERRAIN

In-Office assessment for Sub-clinical hypothyroidism

Hypothyroidism is a very common and often undiagnosed condition.

Blood tests are notoriously insensitive to mild or borderline cases. It has been estimated that based on blood levels of thyroid hormone 1-4% of the US population has moderate to severe hypothyroidism and 10% has mild or borderline hypothyroidism.

In many cases blood levels may be within normal limits yet the patient is suffering from all the classic signs and symptoms of low thyroid.

In these cases it is often more efficacious to look at more functional criteria such as basal body temperature, Achilles return reflex and iodine status, along with history and signs and symptoms.

What causes hypothyroidism?

Hypothyroidism often runs in families. It is more common in females and can be triggered by stress and stressful events such as pregnancy or physical trauma.

Female offspring are more likely to be hypothyroid if their parents or grandparents have been diagnosed with hypothyroidism.

Suspected causes of hypothyroidism

1. Consumption of goitrogens i.e. substances in food that inhibit the normal function of the thyroid and thyroid hormone. Common goitrogens include: sweet potato, cabbage, turnips, rutabagas, peanuts, pine nuts, mustard, millet and soybeans.

2. Iodine insufficiency. Iodine is essential for thyroid hormone production

3. Genetics

4. Environmental pollution. It is well documented that radioactive isotopes have an enormous detrimental impact on the thyroid gland.

5. Heavy metals. Mercury amalgams and prolonged exposure to mercury vapor can have a dramatic impact on thyroid function

NOTES:

6. Chlorine and fluoride in the water. Chlorine, iodine and fluoride belong to the halogen family of elements. Chlorine and fluoride can displace iodine from the body causing thyroid abnormalities.

7. Problems of converting the inactive T4 into the active T3 in the peripheral tissue (Wilson's syndrome)

8. Starvation dieting can cause dramatic swings in the metabolism, which puts stress on the thyroid.

9. Physical or emotional stress

Signs and symptoms of hypothyroidism

- Constipation
- Weight gain with decreased food intake
- Cold intolerance
- Poor circulation
- Fluid retention
- Ringing in the ears

- Poor memory
- Fatigue
- Dry skin and hair
- Hair loss
- Broken nails
- Slow thinking

Laboratory values and hypothyroidism

- Certain lab values may be also be altered with hypothyroidism.

- Complete blood counts may show anemia;

- Chemistry screens may show elevated serum cholesterol;

- Thyroid panels may show decreased T3 uptake, total T4 and free T4 with elevated TSH.

- As mentioned above many patients may not exhibit any laboratory changes, but will have low basal body temperature readings.

NOTES:

Diagnosis

To make an accurate diagnosis of hypothyroidism it is important to include the following:

1. A thorough history, which includes an assessment of all the signs and symptoms of hypothyroidism

2. A blood chemistry analysis, which includes TSH, T4 and free T3, cholesterol, blood glucose, and triglycerides

3. A complete functional physical examination including:

    Achilles return reflex

    Body Temperature Testing

    Iodine Patch test

Achilles return reflex

*   A delayed Achilles return reflex is a classic sign of hypothyroidism.

*   In the absence of spinal lesions, a delayed Achilles return reflex bilaterally indicates the strong likelihood for low thyroid activity, along with the corresponding signs and symptoms.

Body Temperature Test

*   The basal body temperature (BBT) reflects the body's basal metabolism, which refers to the amount of energy your body burns at rest.

*   The basal metabolism is largely determined by hormones secreted from the thyroid and to a lesser degree the adrenal glands.

*   The function of the thyroid can be observed by measuring the fluctuations of the basal body temperature over a number of days.

*   To accurately assess the basal body temperature, a glass, mercury filled thermometer must be used. A special BBT thermometer, available from pharmacies, is more accurate than the common fever thermometers.

*   Temperatures are assessed both under the arm, which more closely correlates with the temperature of the thyroid, and orally.

*   This allows for adrenal and blood sugar fluctuations function to be taken into consideration.

NOTES:

Iodine Patch test

- The iodine Patch test is a functional assessment for iodine status in the body.

- By painting the skin with a 2% solution of iodine we can see how quickly the body absorbs the available iodine.

- If there is a deficiency or need for iodine the slightly brownish yellow patch will fade in less than 24 hours.

- This indicates that there is not sufficient enough iodine to normalize thyroid secretions.

- The quicker the iodine fades, the greater the deficiency can be assumed to be.

NOTES:

ACHILLES RETURN REFLEX

Discussion

 In the absence of spinal lesions a bilateral delay in the Achilles return reflex is a strong indication for low thyroid activity.

It is possible to get a special device that measures the Achilles return speed (Achilliometer), but accurate readings can easily be obtained with practice.

If the patient has brisk Achilles return reflexes and they have symptoms of low thyroid function, consider looking for other causes for their symptoms before treating the thyroid.

When would you run this test?

- To assess for sub clinical hypothyroidism

Directions

1. Have patient kneel or lie with the foot dangling over the edge of the table or chair

2. Tap the tendon directly, with your left hand dorsiflexing the foot for optimal stretching of the tendon

3. As you tap the tendon, the foot should plantar flex briskly, without any delay

Results

Normal: Brisk return of the Achilles reflex bilaterally

Delayed reflex bilaterally: Suspect hypothyroidism

Interfering factors

Neurological deficits e.g. spinal lesions

Related tests

1. Iodine Patch test,

NOTES:

2. Thyroid panel on blood chemistry screen. Please see our book *"Blood Chemistry and CBC Analysis- Clinical Laboratory Testing from a Functional Perspective"* for more details.

3. Body Temperature Test

NOTES:

BODY TEMPERATURE TEST

It is well known that body temperature closely reflects an individual's metabolic energy state. The optimal average day time temperature is 98.6°F. A temperature below that reflects a less than optimal metabolic state.

From our previous discussions we know that a lower than optimal metabolic state is most often controlled at the level of the thyroid, but the adrenals have a hand in it too.

Body temperature can be used diagnostically to check the level of metabolic activity and can be used to monitor treatment.

This is a great tool since it doesn't cost anything and gives patients instant feedback.

If you put a patient on a protocol to correct imbalances seen in the metabolic energy states you can quickly see if the protocol is working. ideally you should see a stable and gradual rise from low and /or unstable temperatures to an optimal 98.6°F.

As you will below, unstable temperatures i.e. a wide variability in body temperature from day to day is a reflection of a weak or fatigued adrenal system.

When would you run this test?

1. To assess the hormonal influences on metabolism

2. To help identify sub clinical hypothyroidism

3. To identify adrenal and blood sugar influences on basal metabolism

Taking and Plotting Temperatures

- The best tool to monitor metabolic changes is a simple thermometer and a temperature graph (see below).

- Temperatures are measured orally because underarm or axillary temperatures are cooler than oral temperatures and tend to be variable in adrenal stress. Taking temperatures by ear is the least reliable. I recommend good old fashioned oral temps.

- In order for the temperature to be accurate you must explain to your patients that they need to place the thermometer deep under the tongue.

- They should avoid taking temperatures after activity (even climbing up stairs can alter the temperature), eating, or drinking for at least 20 minutes.

NOTES:

- I recommend that they take 3 temperatures across the day approximately 3 hours apart. They should take their first morning temperature approximately 3 hours <u>after</u> waking up.

- If your patient rises at 7:30 AM, their temperatures should be taken at 10:30 AM, 1:30 PM, and 5:30 PM. It is best to ask them not to take a number of temperatures in a row because experience shows that the temperature will rise with each subsequent reading.

- Something as simple as the movement of muscles in the mouth can raise the temperature! So it is recommended that your patients take one temperature reading 3 times/day.

What kind of thermometer do you recommend?

- There are a number of excellent models available at your local drug store. You can either purchase a number of them and rent or lend them to your patients, or just make a recommendation of a brand you have tried, is accurate, and gives a quick reading.

- You may want to look at the Lumiscope Digital thermometer. Sadly mercury thermometers are not the most ideal. I say sadly because they are extremely accurate but they contain mercury, can break, are too slow, and if you want to get reproducible temperatures a mercury thermometer must be left in the mouth for the same length of time each time you take a temperature.

Directions of how best to take temperatures:

- Take 3 temperatures a day 3 hours apart from one another.

- Take the first temperature approximately 3 hours after getting up

- Avoid activity, eating, and drinking 20 minutes prior to testing

- Use a digital thermometer, not a mercury or an ear thermometer

- Take only one reading each time

- Fill out the temperature chart and bring it back to the clinic at the next appointment

Recording Temperatures on a Graph

- Have your patients calculate the average of the 3 daily temperatures taken.

- The daily average is then plotted on the graph.

NOTES:

- They can use an X but I recommend that they use a number that represents the number of temperatures taken that day.

- Thus if they only took 2 temperatures on one day they put a number 2 in the cell that corresponds to the average daily temperature and the day of the week the temperature was taken.

- They can also put in additional data such as mood, energy level, changes in supplement protocols or medication etc. This can be helpful when a temperature is out of the usual pattern.

- Finally have them connect the numbers in a line so you get a graphical representation of the temperatures. If they miss a day have them stop and restart the line.

- Do not have them connect the days either side of the missing day.

Interpreting The Temperature Graph

There are some very distinct patterns you can see on a temperature graph:

Stable but low temperatures on graph

- Patients with a **low functioning thyroid or hypothyroidism** typically have very stable, but low temperatures. The graph in this situation will be low but the actual temperature will not vary from day to day. A stable pattern is also seen in healthy individuals. In these cases the temperatures will be at 98.6

Considerable variability and instability on graph- Sharp and Spiky

- Adrenal types i.e. people with **low adrenal function or adrenal fatigue** show considerable variability and instability in their temperatures. Adrenal types are hot in the heat and cold in the cold. This can produce a very unstable pattern. Values may fluctuate from low 98s to low 96s from day to day. The pattern looks very sharp and spiky.

- As your adrenal patients begin to heal you may notice a pattern of contraction in their highs and lows i.e. the differences between their highs and lows are not as extreme. **This is a sign that healing is taking place** and shows stabilization in the pattern. This may be due to either a reduction in stress i.e. a stressful burden has been lifted or there is less thyroid stimulation, or they are getting stronger because of a protocol they are on.

NOTES:

Rising in average temperatures on graph- stable or unstable

- **As the metabolic energy increases** in your patients you may notice a rising in the average temperatures on the graph. The pattern may be stable or unstable.

Increase in variability- an expansion pattern

- You may also note an increase in variability that can be described as an expansion pattern.

- **Greater stress on the adrenals** or an **increase in thyroid stimulation** causes the temperatures to be less stable. This pattern shows that the patient is unable to handle the increasing stress on the body.

- The pattern may be transient i.e. a one off stressful event (a short term increase in workload) or prolonged showing a movement towards maladaptation and worsening adrenal fatigue.

- The thyroid can contribute to this and you will often see this when patients are on T3 therapy and are on a dose that they cannot handle.

A contracting/Rising pattern – a sign of improvement

- A sign that a patient is improving is a contracting/rising pattern. The highs and lows are getting closer together and there is a general rise in body temperature.

NOTE: A sudden rise in temperature lasting one or more days is a sign of an infection producing a fever in the body.

Using the Graph to Monitor Thyroid Therapy

- In a thyroid case the baseline temperatures are going to be low. This may be as low as 96.5°F. The low temperature is typically stable.

- When thyroid therapy (either supplements or armor thyroid) is started you will see a rising pattern in the graph. This is often seen after starting or increasing therapy.

- A pattern that has plateaued and is stable is a sign that the current dose of therapy has taken the body to a particular level of metabolic activity.

- If the plateau is below 98.6°F you may want to increase the dosage of medication. When the therapy has brought the temperature up to 98.6°F and the pattern is stable you know that the correct level of medication has been reached.

NOTES:

- However, you may have reached a level of thyroid support that has taken the body to a level of metabolic energy that is too much for the adrenals to handle. In this situation don't be surprised to see an expansion pattern with a concomitant drop in temperatures.

- This is a good time to look at adrenal support to allow the body to better handle an increase in metabolic activity.

Using the Graph to Monitor Adrenal Therapy

- A baseline pattern of a patient in adrenal fatigue will be the unstable pattern as mentioned above.

- The temperatures are typically below 98.6°F but can fluctuate from day to day, with highs in the low 98s and lows in the 96°F range.

- The temperatures will rise in warm or hot weather and drop in cold or cool weather.

- When adrenal support is started you will notice a decrease in variability and a contraction in the pattern. The highs are not as high and the lows are not as low.

- As adrenal function improves we actually see a stabilization of the pattern but temperatures remain low. This is a good sign.

- The first sign that your adrenal support is working will be the reduction in variability in the temperatures. Continued adrenal support will cause a stabilization in the pattern followed by a gradual rise towards an optimal temperature of 98.6°F, which is a hallmark of a healthy metabolic state.

A Question of Timing

If the adrenal support is working well you should expect to get to the rising stable pattern after a few months. This is of course entirely dependent on how long the adrenal fatigue has been a problem. If the fatigue is severe and chronic each of the above phases may last longer, so you might see it take a month for the variability to reduce, a month for the temperatures to stabilize and start to rise, and another month for the optimal temperature to be achieved.

If you see no response or change in the pattern after a couple of months you may need to change the protocol or consider some other cause, i.e. the patient may be suffering from toxicity.

NOTES:

Related tests

- Iodine Patch test,

- Thyroid panel on blood chemistry screen,

- Achilles return reflex

Form Download

Please download a master copy of my Body Temperature Testing chart at this link:

http://www.BloodChemistryAnalysis.com/pdf files/basal_metabolic_graph.pdf

NOTES:

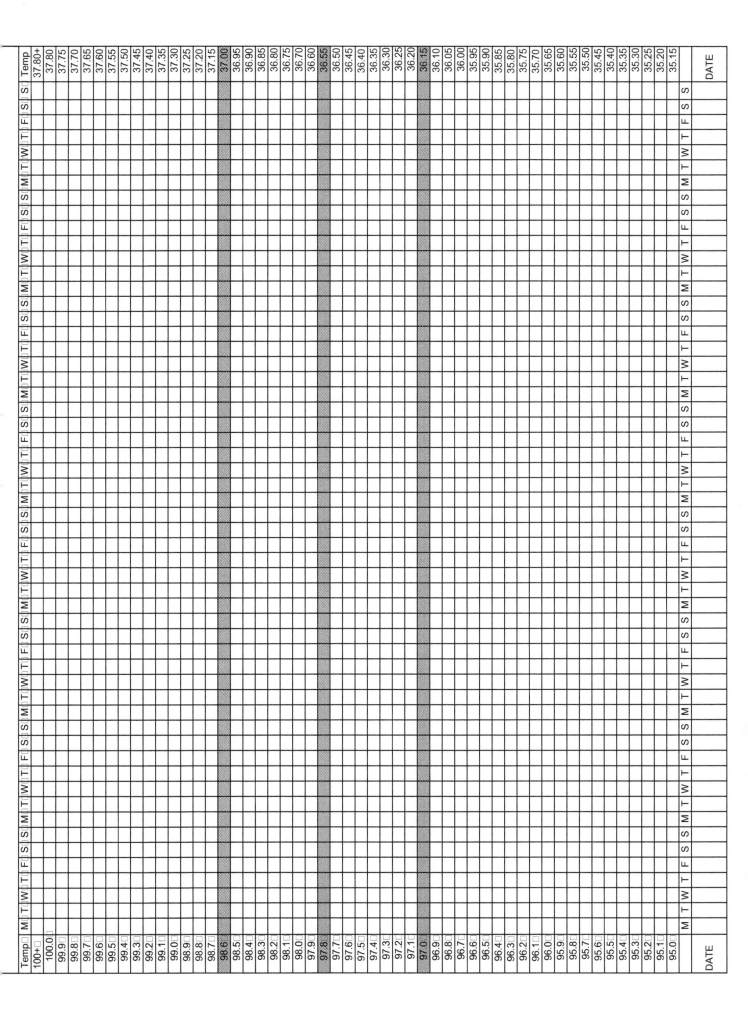

NOTES:

Body Temperature Test Instructions

Name:_____ Date:_____

Your body temperature reflects your metabolism, which is largely determined by the hormones secreted by the thyroid and to a lesser degree, the adrenal glands. Although blood hormone testing is common, there is considerable evidence that the current tests for the diagnosis of hypothyroidism (low thyroid function) are insensitive and somewhat lacking in accuracy. With adrenal function taken into consideration, the function of the thyroid gland can be observed by simply measuring your body temperature. All that is needed is a thermometer.

Instructions:

1. Please measure your temperature orally and place the thermometer deep under your tongue. Do not take your temperature underarm or use an ear thermometer.

2. Avoid taking temperatures after activity (even climbing up stairs can alter the temperature), eating, or drinking for at least 20 minutes.

3. Take 3 temperatures across the day approximately 3 hours apart.

4. Take your first morning temperature approximately 3 hours <u>after</u> waking up i.e. if you rise at 7:30 AM, your temperatures should be taken at 10:30 AM, 1:30 PM, and 5:30 PM. Please do not take a number of temperatures in a row because experience shows that the temperature will rise with each subsequent reading.

What kind of thermometer do you recommend?

There are a number of excellent models available at your local drug store. We recommend the Lumiscope Digital thermometer.

Summary

- Take 3 temperatures a day 3 hours apart from one another.

- Take the first temperature approximately 3 hours after getting up

- Avoid activity, eating, and drinking 20 minutes prior to testing

- Use a digital thermometer, not a mercury or an ear thermometer

- Take only one reading each time

- Fill out the temperature chart and bring it back to the clinic at the next appointment

Recording Temperatures on a Graph

- Please calculate the average of the 3 daily temperatures taken and plot that average on the graph.

- We recommend that you use a number that represents the number of temperatures taken that day when writing on the graph.

- Thus if you only took 2 temperatures on one day you put a number 2 in the cell that corresponds to the average daily temperature and the day of the week the temperature was taken.

- You can also put in additional data such as mood, energy level, changes in supplement protocols or medication etc. This can be helpful for us to work out the pattern of the temperature changes.

- Finally please connect the numbers in a line so we get a graphical representation of the temperatures. If you miss a day please stop and restart the line i.e. do not connect the days either side of the missing day.

- Please plot your averages on the graph on the next page.

NOTES:

IODINE PATCH TEST

Discussion

 Iodine is a nutrient that is deficient in many people. It is essential for thyroid function, being an integral part of the thyroxine molecule.

The iodine patch test is a functional assessment for iodine status in the body. By painting the skin with a 2% solution of iodine we can see how quickly the body absorbs the available iodine.

If there is a deficiency or need for iodine the slightly brownish yellow stain will fade in less than 24 hours. This indicates that there is not sufficient enough iodine to normalize thyroid secretions. The quicker the iodine fades, the greater the deficiency can be assumed to be.

Functions of Iodine

- Principal role in the manufacturer of thyroid hormone

- Modulation of the effect of estrogen on breast tissue

- The conversion of estrone and estradiol into estriol

Results

Color lasts for > 24 hours   Sufficient iodine

Color fades in < 24 hours   Deficient iodine

When would you run this test?

1. When iodine deficiency is suspected

2. Patients present with signs of hypothyroidism

3. Patients with low basal body temperatures

NOTES:

Clinical implications

As was mentioned above, the quicker the iodine fades, the greater the deficiency can be assumed to be. The following protocol should be implemented until sufficiency is obtained i.e. the stain remains for a minimum of 24 hours:

20-30 drops of liquid iodine (as potassium iodide) per day

Interfering Factors

Patients may react to the topical application of iodine or they may present with symptoms of iodism (too much iodine), which are tachycardia, skin irritation, thinning of secretions (watery eyes, nose, saliva), nervousness and headache.

Related Tests

- Body Temperature Test

- Blood Chemistries: thyroid panel. Please see our book *"Blood Chemistry and CBC Analysis- Clinical Laboratory Testing from a Functional Perspective"* for more details.

- Achilles Return Reflex

NOTES:

HYPOADRENALISM VS. HYPOTHYROIDISM

As mentioned above, hypoadrenalism has a number of overlapping symptoms with hypothyroidism. Low thyroid and low adrenals both produce low body temperature and low metabolic states and they share many of the same symptoms:

- Slow healing

- Weakened system

- Low physical and mental energy

- Cold hands and feet

Other symptoms are quite the opposite of each other. This is especially important when treating the thyroid does not improve the symptoms. In these cases think that hypoadrenalism may be the issue.

The following tables represent some of the basic differences in terms of signs and symptoms and physical exam findings.

Signs and Symptoms

S/SX	ADRENAL	THYROID
Body type	Thin, cannot gain weight	Cannot lose weight
Temperature	Thermal changing: hot when it is hot, cold when cold. Tends to low body temperature around 97.8	Stable, non-fluctuating but low. Can range from 98.4 (mild) to 95.0 (severe)
Tolerance to stress	Poor	Moderate
Hair quality	Thin and wispy	Coarse
Skin	Dry and thin	Poor healing
Body water	Tendency to dryness	Fluid retention
Blood sugar	Hypoglycemia	Normal to hyperglycemia
Blood pressure	Tends to run low	Normal to high

NOTES:

Findings on Physical Exam

PE	ADRENAL	THYROID
Pupillary constriction	Usually under 5 seconds	Usually over 5 seconds
Tissue around eyes	Sunken appearance	Puffy around eyes
Weight distribution	Uniformly thin	Uniformly heavy or more in low body
Edema (non-pitting)	-	++
Reflexes	-	+
Heart: mitral valve problems	+/++	-
Hair: thin on arms and/or absent on legs	++	-

Acid – Alkaline Terrain

NOTES:

ACID – ALKALINE TERRAIN

Acid-Alkaline balance and its impact on the Terrain

One of the conditions that causes the internal terrain to drift away from optimal is an imbalance in the acid and alkaline or pH system. It is important to remember that we are talking about functional imbalances in the acid/alkaline system, and not the pathological variances in pH that are often seen in the emergency room. The terms acidosis and alkalosis are often used indiscriminately. Acidosis, for instance, is blamed for many of the ills of modern living. These claims are made without a true appreciation for acid/alkaline biochemistry or physiology.

In this section we will discuss how the biochemistry and physiology of pH can be applied clinically, we will discuss the primary and secondary methods that the body uses to maintain optimal pH and the patterns of acid/alkaline imbalance that can arise when these methods of pH control become compromised. We will teach you the in-office tests that can help determine exactly whether a primary acid/alkaline imbalance exists, and methods for assessing imbalances in the secondary compensatory systems.

A balanced acid-alkaline system is important for the following reasons:

- Even a slight variation of pH from optimal will have wide reaching impacts on the body. For instance the blood has a pH range of 7.35 to 7.45 that needs to be very tightly regulated. If the pH of the blood were to drop to 6.95, coma and death would follow!

- A balanced pH is essential for the thousands of enzymes and other chemical reactions that happen within the body.

- Hormone levels fluctuate when there is an imbalance in the pH. For example, levels of hormones like epinephrine and aldosterone will increase as the body becomes more acid.

- Hemoglobin's ability to carry and release oxygen and carbon dioxide will vary depending on the pH of the blood.

- Blood sugar regulation requires a balanced pH. The ability of the cell to recognize insulin is greatly affected by pH fluctuations.

- Changes in intracellular and extracellular pH have a profound effect on the mineral reserves in the body, which act as short-term buffers.

NOTES:

- The digestive system functions in a very specific pH range. The stomach requires a very acidic pH, whereas the pancreas requires an alkaline pH.

- Every cell needs a balanced ph for the movement of nutrients into the cell and metabolic waste and toxicity out of the cell.

- Glycolosis, the Kreb's cycle and oxidative phosphorylation, the energy producing systems of the body, require a balanced pH for optimal production of ATP

What are the pH ranges found in the various fluids and tissues in the body?

BODY FLUIDS and TISSUE	pH
Saliva	6.0-7.4
Food entering stomach	5.0-6.0
Stomach secretions	1.5-4.0
Digestive secretions from liver and liver bile	7.1-8.5
Bile from gallbladder	5.0-7.7
Pancreatic and biliary secretions into small intestine	7.5-8.3
Urine	4.5-8.0
Blood	7.35-7.45

- With the exception of the blood the majority of fluids in the body have wide pH ranges, which exist so that these fluids can shift their pH to maintain the balance of blood pH.

- With the exception of the stomach, the body fluids are all alkaline. The body functions best when the pH of these tissues and fluids are kept within an optimal range.

- Imbalances in the acid-alkaline terrain occur when these optimal pH levels are not maintained.

NOTES:

What are the effects of acid/alkaline imbalance in the body?

1. **Enzyme systems in the body fail to work**. There are thousands of enzyme reactions taking place in our bodies every second. Each of these reactions is like a complex key that needs to "fit" into a specific keyhole. If blood pH is off balance even a little, some important keys are not "fitting" their respective slots. Enzyme function and the essential chemical reactions they facilitate begin to suffer.

2. **The oxygen delivery mechanisms in the blood become compromised**. The body stores excess acidity in the extracellular matrix (the spaces around the cells) of the tissues. The blood, in order to compensate for this, becomes increasingly alkaline. With rising alkalinity, the red blood cells can saturate themselves in oxygen. Increasing oxygen saturation seems like a good thing, until you realize that the major problem is the red blood cells cannot release the oxygen. If the blood cells cannot let go of the oxygen, then the oxygen isn't getting into the cells of the body leading to tissue hypoxia and decreased production of ATP. It is becoming clearer from research that low oxygen delivery to cells is a major factor in most if not all degenerative conditions, and it is well known that cancer grows in an oxygen deficient environment.

3. **Blood sugar dysregulation:** Insulin facilitates the movement of glucose into the cell. The ability of the cells to recognize insulin is greatly affected by pH fluctuations in the blood. The brain is one organ that is especially vulnerable to this phenomenon because it cannot store glucose and as such relies on the second to second supply of glucose from the bloodstream. pH fluctuations in the blood are perhaps one of the reasons for much of the blood sugar dysregulation seen today.

4. **Digestive function becomes compromised.** Pancreatic insufficiency is influenced by the body using alkaline pancreatic juices to buffer an acidic blood. Hypochlorhydria is influenced by the body using acidic stomach secretions to buffer an alkaline blood.

5. **Electrolyte and mineral imbalance.** A catch-22 situation occurs in the body when the pH of the blood begins to drift. As we have seen above the body uses alkaline minerals and digestive juices to buffer the blood. Unfortunately the use of the digestive juices to buffer the blood leads to less than optimal digestion, which has a profound effect on the digestion, absorption and assimilation of the alkaline minerals that the body uses to buffer the blood! The availability of these essential electrolytes and minerals is compromised, causing an electrolyte and mineral imbalance. Acids bind up the minerals in the buffering system and they are no longer available to act as the co-factors for the thousands of mineral dependent enzyme reactions. An electrolyte imbalance will have an effect on the ability of both the extracellular fluid to carry nutrients and waste in and out of the cell, and the cell to carry on oxidation and other essential metabolic processes.

NOTES:

6. **The electrical potential of the cell begins to change.** pH imbalances in the extracellular fluids interferes with the potential energy of the cell. The electrical cell potential is usually between −70 to -90mV, which is the optimal range for the movement of nutrients into the cell and waste products out of the cell. Hyperacidity, heavy metals in the extracellular matrix and possibly electromagnetic stress from microwaves and cellular phones drop the voltage as low as 0mV. Under these circumstances, the cells are no longer able to remove waste. Instead they store waste, which greatly reduces their function. As cellular function becomes compromised so does the production of ATP.

How does the body maintain optimal pH?

- The body uses a number of complex buffering systems to keep pH within a normal and optimal range.

1° Buffering System	2° Buffering Systems
• Bicarbonate buffering system (lungs and kidneys)	• Alkaline minerals • Urea cycle (liver) and ammonia • Digestive system
The system used for about 90% of acid/alkaline buffering	The systems used for about 10% of acid/alkaline buffering

NOTES:

PRIMARY BUFFERING SYSTEM

Bicarbonate Buffering System

The bicarbonate buffering system is the primary extracellular buffering system of the body. Intracellular and plasma buffering is mostly handled by powerful protein buffers. In this section we will look at the following:

- The biochemistry and physiology that underlies the bicarbonate buffering system.

- The patterns of acid/alkaline imbalance that occur when this system of pH compensation is compromised.

- The clinical tests that can be used to determine if a pattern of imbalance exists, and what the specific imbalance is.

The bicarbonate buffering system is the primary extracellular buffer in the body. It accounts for about 90% of the body's extracellular pH buffering. In this system, carbon dioxide, an acidic by-product of oxidative phosphorylation, combines with water using an enzyme called carbonic anhydrase, (an enzyme that needs the mineral zinc as a co-enzyme), to form carbonic acid. Carbonic acid is fairly unstable in solution and will dissociate into its ionic form of a bicarbonate ion and a hydrogen ion:

$$CO_2 \quad + H_2O \quad \Leftrightarrow \quad H_2CO_3 \quad \Leftrightarrow \quad HCO_3^- \quad + H^+$$

Carbon Dioxide	Water	Carbonic acid	Bicarbonate ion	Hydrogen ion

An increase in dissolved CO_2 will decrease the pH, or shift the acid-alkaline balance to the acid side.

An increase of bicarbonate ion concentration will cause the pH to rise i.e. shift to the alkaline side.

- The bicarbonate buffering system is not a closed one, because the body is constantly losing CO_2 through respiration and bicarbonate and H+ through the kidneys. The body, therefore, has to use the respiratory and renal systems to control pH fluctuations.

NOTES:

The Respiratory system: Alteration of the respiration rate and depth of breathing to control pH

The body uses alterations in the respiration rate and depth of breathing to change the relative concentration of CO_2 in the blood and therefore control pH fluctuations:

- By increasing the respiration rate i.e. through hyperventilation, more CO_2 is expelled from the body, which in turn raises the pH (more alkaline)

- By decreasing the respiration rate i.e. through hypoventilation, less CO_2 is expelled from the body, which lowers the pH (more acidic)

The respiratory system accounts for 50%-70% of pH compensation, when the Bicarbonate buffering system is used.

Renal system: Alterations in the kidneys ability to reabsorb or excrete bicarbonate and H+

The body uses the kidney's ability to reabsorb or excrete bicarbonate and H+ to change the relative concentration of bicarbonate or H+ in the blood. The kidney, in collaboration with the liver, uses the following mechanisms:

- Increased reabsorption of bicarbonate by the kidney in the descending loop of Henle will increase blood bicarbonate and thus raise the pH (more alkaline)

- Decreased reabsorption or increased excretion of bicarbonate will decrease blood bicarbonate and thus lower the pH (more acidic)

The renal system accounts for 30%-50% of pH compensation, when the primary bicarbonate buffering system is used.

NOTES:

What are some of the patterns of acid/alkaline imbalance?

Factors outside of the body's control can begin to alter the body's pH. There are four main patterns of acid/alkaline imbalance that are seen when this happens:

1. Metabolic acidosis 2. Metabolic alkalosis	3. Respiratory acidosis 4. Respiratory Alkalosis
• Two patterns of acid/base imbalance that are caused by alterations in bicarbonate (HCO_3^-) or H+ concentrations	• Two patterns of acid/base imbalance caused by alterations in CO_2 concentrations

In these situations, the bicarbonate buffer begins to compensate:

- The body begins to alter the respiration rate and depth of breathing in order to compensate by lowering or raising the amount of dissolved CO^2

- The body begins to alter the reabsorption or excretion of either bicarbonate ($HCO3^-$) or H+

Clinical determination of patterns of acid/alkaline imbalance

When we are making a clinical determination of an acid/alkaline imbalance, we are measuring the body's compensatory mechanisms at work. It is important to remember the following:

- Acid/alkaline imbalances in the bicarbonate buffering system **always** involve the respiratory functions

- Acid/alkaline imbalances in the bicarbonate buffering system **always** involve the kidneys.

It is also important to remember to ask yourself whether you are looking at the primary cause of the problem or the body's defense or compensation. This is most easily seen in respiratory system, which is always associated with an acidosis or alkalosis.

The respiratory system can be the primary cause of the imbalance, or, it can be the primary defense in compensation for the imbalance. Whether as cause or an effect, the respiratory system is always part of the clinical picture in evaluating the patterns of acid/alkaline imbalance in the bicarbonate buffering system.

NOTES:

Respiratory system as a 1° cause of acid/alkaline imbalance		Respiratory system as a compensation for acid/alkaline imbalance	
• Causative in Respiratory acidosis and Respiratory alkalosis		• Compensatory in Metabolic acidosis and Metabolic alkalosis	
Respiratory acidosis	• Caused by hypoventilation • CO_2 produced faster than it can be blown off • ↑ carbonic acid retention → acidosis	**Metabolic acidosis**	• Respiratory activity is increased • CO_2 blown off to lower carbonic acid levels
Respiratory alkalosis	• Caused by hyperventilation • CO_2 blown off faster than it can be produced • ↓ carbonic acid levels→, alkalosis.	**Metabolic alkalosis**	• Respiratory activity slowed down • Retention of CO_2 in the form of carbonic acid to decrease the alkalosis.

NOTES:

CLINICAL ASSESSMENT OF ACID/ALKALINE IMBALANCES

Given the above information the best way to make clinical assessments of acid/alkaline imbalances is to observe the patterns between the following:

1. Breath holding time

2. Respiration rate

3. Urine pH

4. Saliva pH

Breath holding time and respiration rate

Breath holding time and respiration rate are used to measure the involvement of the respiratory system in patterns of acid/alkaline imbalance in the bicarbonate buffering system.

Since the respiratory system accounts for 50%-70% of pH compensation, the breath holding time and the respiration rate are the main tests used to indicate the **presence** of an acidosis or alkalosis.

NOTE: If your patient has a normal breath hold time and respiration rate then there is *no* imbalance in the primary buffering system

Urine pH and Salivary pH

The urine pH and salivary pH are used to help identify the **type** of acidosis or alkalosis, but not the presence of acidosis or alkalosis—only the breath hold time and respiration do that.

The following section will go into more detail on the specific patterns of acid/alkaline imbalance, the clinical findings associated with each imbalance, and the causes and the signs and symptoms of acidosis and alkalosis.

NOTES:

BREATH – HOLD TEST

Discussion

In the absence of cardiovascular, pulmonary or respiratory tract infections, breath-holding time reflects acid/alkaline imbalance.

- In an acidosis there is a decreased transport and uptake of oxygen by the body, which leads to a decreased breath holding time.

- In an alkalosis there is a slight increased uptake and transport of oxygen, as well as a compensatory suppression of the respiratory center, which leads to the ability to hold ones breath longer.

When would you run this test?

- To check a patient for acid/alkaline imbalance

Directions

This test is an actual measurement of how long the patient can hold a deep breath. With the patient sitting, ask them to "take a deep breath and hold it as long as you can". Use a stopwatch or timer to time the breath holding. When the patient can no longer hold their breath, record the seconds the breath was held on the results form.

Results

Normal: 40-65 seconds

Clinical implications

INCREASED BREATH-HOLD TIME

Clinical Implication	Additional information
Metabolic alkalosis **Respiratory alkalosis**	Alkalosis causes an increased oxygen uptake and transport leading to an increased ability to hold ones breath

NOTES:

DECREASED BREATH-HOLD TIME

Clinical Implication	Additional information
Metabolic acidosis **Respiratory acidosis**	In acidosis a decreased transport and uptake of oxygen by the body leads to a decreased breath holding time.
Anemia	Decreased oxygen-carrying capacity of red-blood cells due to anemia may decrease breath-hold time
Other causes include:	Antioxidant deficiency, emotional stress, anxiety

Interfering Factors

Cardio-pulmonary disease, respiratory tract infections

NOTES:

RESPIRATORY RATE

Discussion

 Respiratory rate is used in determining acid/alkaline imbalances in your patients. The respiratory rate is set from the respiratory centers in the brain and responds to oxygen saturation of blood that flows through the aortic and carotid arteries.

When would you run this test?

- To check a patient for acid/alkaline imbalance

Directions

- This test is a measurement of respiratory rate. It is best not to tell the patient that you are going to take a respiratory rate because they will invariably alter their breathing rate and skew the results.

- The best method of taking a respiratory rate is to tell patient that you are going to take a pulse for one minute and count the pulse for the first 30 seconds and the respiratory rate for the latter 30 seconds.

- Using a stopwatch, a timer or a watch with a second-hand, hold the patient's wrist and gently place your hand on the upper abdomen and count the pulse and the number of respiratory cycles in 30 seconds. Multiply by two and record the number on the results form.

Results

Normal: 14-18 respiratory cycles/minute

Clinical implications

INCREASED RESPIRATORY RATE (hyperventilation)

Clinical Implication	Additional information
Metabolic acidosis	In metabolic acidosis the body increases respiratory rate as a means of blowing off CO_2 and thus lowering carbonic acid levels and relieve the acidosis.

NOTES:

Clinical Implication	Additional information
Respiratory acidosis (compensation)	The increased respiratory rate is a sign of compensation by the body in dealing with respiratory acidosis, which has an etiology in hypoventilation i.e. CO_2 levels increase because the body is unable to blow it off (e.g. in asthma and emphysema). The increased respiration rate is the body's way of compensating. The breathing is rapid and often shallow.
Respiratory alkalosis (Primary cause/acute)	Respiratory alkalosis is caused by hyperventilation or an increased respiratory rate. In the acute or primary phase there is hyperventilation, as the body begins to compensate we see the respiration rate decrease
Sympathetic stress	Increased sympathetic output can cause hyperventilation

NOTES:

DECREASED RESPIRATORY RATE

Clinical Implication	Additional information
Metabolic alkalosis	A slowing of the reparation rate is due to the suppression of the respiratory centers (the body is attempting to lessen the amount of CO_2 blown off to increase carbonic acid levels)
Respiratory alkalosis (chronic or compensation/ recovery stage)	Respiratory alkalosis is caused by hyperventilation. The reduced respiratory rate is the body's attempt to counter the alkalosis by slowing the breath and therefore increasing the levels of CO_2 and carbonic acid.
Respiratory acidosis **In primary cause (usually accompanied by high blood pressure)**	As blood pressure increases the aorta and carotid arteries carry more oxygenated blood past the chemoreceptors, which are stimulated and begin to lower the respiratory rate by changing rate and depth of breathing. This can lead to respiratory acidosis.

Interfering Factors

Cardio-pulmonary disease, respiratory tract infections

Related Tests

- Urine pH

- Saliva pH

- Breath-Hold test

NOTES:

URINE PH

Discussion

 The urine pH indicates the efforts of the body via the kidneys, lungs and adrenals to regulate pH through the various buffering systems.

- It also indicates how the body is tolerating the food you eat.

- The acid-alkaline system in the body is not a static process but a dynamic and cyclical one.

- As we go through the day our urine becomes progressively more alkaline. This is a result of the alkaline tide, the body's method of dumping alkalinity to compensate for hydrochloric acid loss during digestion.

- We cannot, therefore make a determination of overall pH of the body just by measuring urine pH once. We need to test samples from across the day, including a sample from the first morning urine and evaluate them with other parameters such as saliva pH, breath holding time and respiration rate.

1st Morning Urine

- The first morning urine is the first urination after 4:00 AM. In an ideal situation where your patients are truly healthy in all aspects of their physiology and biochemistry, the urine pH, after at least five hours sleep, should register around pH 7.0. However, this is not often the case.

- Given the lifestyle that most people lead, the first morning urine should register between 5.4 and 5.65. This may not be the most optimum but it shows that the body is compensating well.

- The urine is very acidic due to the prior hours of fasting during sleep, the mild respiratory acidosis, caused by decreased pulmonary ventilation, and the metabolic acids filtered and processed by the kidneys and accumulated by the bladder during the night.

- The pH of the first morning sample is used only as a reference for subsequent samples. It will be used in almost all of the other metabolic urine tests.

Subsequent Urine samples

- As we start the day, we begin to breath more normally, to digest food and release the acid reserves. The respiratory acidosis begins to diminish and we

NOTES:

get some alkaline buffering from HCl secretion in the gastric juices. All of this causes the urine to become more alkaline. The urine should ideally be between 6.4 and 6.8.

- Many people tend to stay too acidic (urine pH < than 6.4), while fewer are more alkaline (higher pH > 6.7). Of the two, it's better to be more acidic than alkaline because the body has more buffering systems to handle excess acidity than excess alkalinity.

- Please use this sample in making pH assessments in relation to saliva pH, breath hold time and respiration rate.

Urine sample collection times

To get an accurate assessment of the body's pH system we recommend the following:

- Test the pH of the first morning urination after 4:00 AM

- Test the pH of the second morning urination

- If at all possible test the pH of the urine at the office visit

- Please retain the first morning urine because you will be doing most of your metabolic urinalysis on this sample.

NOTE: All urine should be refrigerated after it has been collected, and stored in the refrigerator in your office

Directions

Although you can get urine pH from a reagent dipstick, you can get a much more accurate reading using an electronic pH meter.

- Remove protective cap on pH meter

- Insert pH meter into urine specimen and obtain digital reading

- Record reading and clean pH meter

- Calibration should take place after every 10-15 tests

When would you run this test?

- To assess for pH imbalances by assessing buffering systems

- To screen for urinary tract infections

NOTES:

Clinical implications

1ST MORNING URINE SAMPLE

Optimum Range

1st morning urine: 5.4-5.65

This sample is used as a reference point for subsequent samples

Urine pH: 5.65-6.8

Clinical Implication	Additional information
Increasing loss of buffer control	The body is not able to fully release stored acids, which indicates a growing difficulty in maintaining buffering control.

Urine pH:>6.8

Clinical Implication	Additional information
Bacterial infection	Alkaline urine is the perfect environment for a urinary tract bacterial infection. Need to rule this out first with a dipstick test for nitrites and leukocyte esterase. Common organisms include Proteus and Pseudomonas
Kidney stress	A symptom of an overly acidic body. The kidney is no longer able to keep up with the free unbuffered acids. It compensates by dumping the alkaline reserves.
Liver stress	Liver support is needed to enhance the urea cycle, which will increase the body's ability to remove excess acids and take the stress off of the kidneys.

NOTES:

SUBSEQUENT URINE SAMPLES

Optimum range

Subsequent samples: 6.4-6.8

The value that should be used in the pH assessments patterns

Alkaline urine- Urine pH: > 6.8

Clinical Implication	Additional information
Bacterial infection	Alkaline urine is the perfect environment for a urinary tract bacterial infection. Need to rule this out first with a dipstick test for nitrites and leukocyte esterase. Common organisms include Proteus and Pseudomonas
Susceptibility to viruses and yeast	People who tend to have an alkaline pH also tend to have more susceptibility to viral conditions, chronic fatigue, Epstein Barr, and Candida (yeast overgrowth).
Protein maldigestion	A patient whose pH is consistently above 6.7 does not digest their proteins optimally due to a protease deficiency
Alkalosis (respiratory or metabolic)	The body responds to an alkalosis by causing the kidney to both retain acid in the form of hydrogen, and to excrete bicarbonate. Both of these will lead to alkaline urine.
Other possible problems of urine pH increase.	Calcium metabolism problems Anxiety Immune dysfunction
These conditions may be associated with an alkaline urine	Pyloric obstruction, salicylate intoxication, renal tubular acidosis, chronic renal failure, respiratory diseases involving hyperventilation and loss of CO_2, vomiting, metabolic alkalosis

NOTES:

Acidic urine- Urine pH < 6.4

Acidic urine indicates an abundance of exogenously or endogenously produced acids, which are being excreted by the kidney.

Clinical Implication	Additional information
Maldigestion	The incomplete oxidation of food, leads to an excess acid production in the tissue that are being excreted
Carbohydrate and fat maldigestion	People, who are consistently acidic (below 6.4 pH), do not optimally digest carbohydrates and fats.
Pancreatic insufficiency	Excess acid reserve means that not enough alkalinity is present to activate pancreatic enzymes in the duodenum.
Acidosis (respiratory and metabolic)	The body responds to an acidosis by causing the kidneys to dump hydrogen and ammonia thus creating acidic urine.
Other problems of a urine pH decrease	Being more prone to acidic, hot, irritating conditions such as inflammation, degeneration, arthritis, and skin irritations.
These conditions may be associated with an acid pH	Metabolic and respiratory acidosis, uncontrolled diabetes, pulmonary emphysema, diarrhea, fasting and starvation, dehydration

NOTES:

Interfering Factors

Falsely increased levels	Falsely decreased levels
• A urine sample that is left to stand, un-refrigerated will become alkaline because bacteria split the urea into ammonia (a base). Urine must be refrigerated if there is a delay between sample collection and testing	• Consumption of cranberry juice may falsely acidify the urine • Ammonium chloride supplementation

Related Tests

- Salivary pH

- Breath holding time

- Respiration rate

- Urinary calcium

- Urinary sediment

- Urinary chloride

NOTES:

SALIVARY pH

Discussion

 Saliva is formed from the same interstitial fluid as the lymph. It contains the following secretions:

- A serous secretion called ptyalin, an alpha amylase, which is a carbohydrate-digesting enzyme,

- Mucous secretions, containing mucin, for lubrication

- Interstitial fluid, which contains alkaline minerals and bicarbonate.

Salivary pH is a fair indicator of the health of the extracellular fluids, their alkaline mineral reserves and, along with parameters such as urine pH, breath holding time and respiration rate, can be used to assess the body's regulation of pH.

- An optimum salivary pH that is slightly alkaline is necessary to provide the correct pH for effective ptyalin activity, a pH dependent enzyme.

- A person with an optimum salivary pH between 7.1 and 7.4 is less likely to be deficient in essential fatty acids.

Salivary pH depends on a number of different physiological parameters:

1. The most important physiological parameter is the relative concentration of free CO_2 and combined CO_2, in the form of carbonic acid (H_2CO_3). This buffering system will have the largest single effect on salivary pH.

- A high CO2 concentration in the blood will cause an increase in carbonic acid, which will cause acidic saliva. This pattern is seen in respiratory acidosis and metabolic alkalosis.

- A low CO2 concentration will cause a decrease in carbonic acid, which in turn will lead to alkaline saliva. This pattern is seen in respiratory alkalosis and metabolic acidosis.

2. The ratio of metabolic acids and alkaline forming electrolytes in the lymph or interstitial fluid will also impact salivary pH.

NOTES:

- The pH of your saliva moves from low to high across the day according to what you eat, how you breathe and how your body is compensating for acid and alkaline shifts.

- It is useful to get the first morning salivary pH as a reference to subsequent samples. Testing a random sample in the office will suffice for making pH determinations.

1st morning salivary sample

In a healthy person the first salivary sample should be slightly acidic at about 6.8. This reflects the mild respiratory acidosis, caused by decreased pulmonary ventilation, and the increased acids that have been built up overnight. Ask your patients to take this pH as a reference point and bring the result into the office with them. You want to see the saliva becoming more alkaline as the day progresses.

Subsequent salivary pH samples

Subsequent salivary pH samples should change toward a slightly alkaline reading of 7.1 -7.4. As the days progresses we begin to breathe more normally and begin to eat. The saliva becomes more alkaline, which provides the correct pH for optimum amylase activity. When there are enough reserves to buffer the acid produced naturally by cellular activity, saliva pH will register around 7.1-7.4. Readings of considerably lower or higher than this usually indicate that the body has alkaline mineral deficiencies and food will not be assimilated very well due to inefficient digestive enzyme activity.

Directions

- Testing must be done at least 30 minutes from any food or beverage.

- Place a pH testing strip in their mouth on top of the tongue. They should get it good and moist.

- Lips must remain closed, as clinical readings of salivary pH must not allow exposure of the sample to air, which can result in inaccurate readings.

- Immediately after removing the pH strip (reading must be made within 3 seconds) compare the strip with the color code on the box.

When would you run this test?

- To assess a patient's acid/alkaline balance

- A good general indicator for carbohydrate digestion

NOTES:

- A good assessment for Essential Fatty Acid (EFA) need

Optimal Ranges

First morning sample: 6.7-6.9

Subsequent samples: 7.1-7.4

Clinical implications

ALKALINE SALIVA

Clinical Implication	Additional information
Metabolic Acidosis	The body responds to an acidosis by causing an increase in respiration to blow off CO_2 and thus lower carbonic acid in the body, which leads to a more alkaline salivary pH.
Respiratory alkalosis	Situation of extreme physiological stress can cause respiratory alkalosis. Too much CO_2 is "blown off" from increased respirations or hyperventilation. This causes alkaline saliva.
Maldigestion	The more alkaline the saliva gets, the weaker the digestive juices in the stomach may become, causing maldigestion
Hypochlorhydria	Alkaline saliva may be another marker for hypochlorhydria, which can upset the gastrointestinal equilibrium causing dysbiosis, yeast etc. that thrive in an abnormal digestive pH.
Sympathetic dominance	Sympathetic dominance causes an increase excretion of potassium, which occurs with increased cellular acidity.
Alkaline Mineral insufficiency	Acidic or alkaline saliva indicates that the alkaline mineral buffering reserves have been depleted and the body is being forced to compensate by other means.
Dental tartar	Alkaline saliva is one of the major causes of tartar build-up on the teeth
Symptoms associated with ↑ saliva pH	Increased respiration, stiff joints, muscle cramps, calcium deposition in soft tissues, hypoglycemia, discomfort after eating, dysbiosis

NOTES:

ACIDIC SALIVA

Clinical Implication	Additional information
Metabolic Alkalosis	The body responds to an alkalosis by causing a compensatory suppression of the respiratory center in an attempt to retain CO_2, which leads to increased levels of carbonic acid, and an acid saliva.
Respiratory acidosis	Respiratory acidosis is due to insufficient respirations or air exchange, which causes increased CO_2 in the blood and a concomitant acidic saliva
Malabsorption	May indicate a decreased bowel transit time as foods are moving too quickly through the digestive tract thus decreasing the absorptive time
Carbohydrate maldigestion	Effective carbohydrate digestion relies on the activation of alpha amylase in the saliva. A salivary pH below 7.1 will not provide the optimum pH for alpha amylase activity, causing possible gas and bloating.
Pancreatic insufficiency	Improper digestion due to lack of enzymes can lead to an increase in metabolic acids which will cause acidity to build up in the interstitial fluids thus affecting salivary pH
Essential fatty acid deficiency	A salivary pH below 7.2 may indicate a deficiency in essential fatty acids.
Fat digestion problems	Excess dietary fats or an inability to completely metabolize fats will cause an increase in ketones, which will increase the acids present in the interstitium.
Alkaline Mineral insufficiency	Alkaline or acidic saliva indicates that the alkaline mineral buffering reserves have been depleted and the body is being forced to compensate by other means.
Dental caries	Acidic saliva is one of the leading causes of dental caries and tooth decay
Other conditions associated with acidic saliva	<table><tr><td>• Anxiety • Chronic stress • Need for detoxification</td><td>• Mental/emotional factors • Lack of exercise</td></tr></table>

NOTES:

Interfering Factors

Falsely increased levels	Falsely decreased levels
• Exercise and perspiration increase saliva pH causing loss of acids through the skin • Increases during meals	• Smoking • Saliva pH decreases during sleep, after meals • Bacteria and microbes in the mouth

Related Tests

- Urine pH,

- Breath-holding time,

- Respiration rate

NOTES:

Clinical Findings In Patterns Of Acidosis And Alkalosis

PATTERN	METABOLIC ACIDOSIS	METABOLIC ALKALOSIS
Discussion	A build-up of H+ in cellular fluids that leads to systemic acidosis	↑ Excretion of H+ or retention of HCO_3^- →systemic alkalosis
Respiration rate	**Increased** The respiratory system compensates by ↑ the rate and depth of respiration to blow off CO_2 and ↓ carbonic acid levels	**Decreased** Suppression of respiratory centers causes ↓ rate and depth of respiration to retain CO_2 and ↑ carbonic acid levels
Breath hold time	**Decreased** Acidosis causes a ↓ O_2 transport and uptake leading to a ↓ ability to hold one's breath	**Increased** Alkalosis causes an ↑ O_2 transport and uptake leading to a ↑ ability to hold one's breath
Urine pH	**Decreased** **Acidic urine-** kidneys compensate by excreting H+ in urine and retaining bicarbonate	**Increased** **Alkaline urine-** Kidneys compensate by retaining H+ and excreting bicarbonate in urine
Saliva pH	**Increased** **Alkaline saliva-** ↑ respiratory rate lowers the dissolved carbonic acid levels resulting in alkaline saliva	**Decreased** **Acidic saliva-** ↓ respiratory rate increases dissolved carbonic acid levels resulting in acidic saliva

PATTERN	RESPIRATORY ACIDOSIS	RESPIRATORY ALKALOSIS
Discussion	Retention of H+ due to ↓ excretion of CO_2 from lungs	Loss of H+ due to ↑ excretion of CO_2 from lungs- hyperventilation
Respiration rate	**Decreased as a 1° cause** ↓ Respiration rate (hypoventilation) is the primary cause of acidosis in respiratory acidosis. **Increased in compensation** The respiration rate is ↑ in respiratory compensation for metabolic acidosis. Rate and depth of respiration is ↑ to blow off more CO_2 and ↓ carbonic acid levels.	**Increased as a 1° cause** ↑ Respiration rate (hyperventilation) is the primary cause of alkalosis in respiratory alkalosis **Decreased in compensation** The respiration rate is ↓ in respiratory compensation for metabolic alkalosis. Rate and depth of respiration is ↓ to retain more CO_2 and ↑ carbonic acid levels.
Breath hold time	**Decreased** Acidosis causes a ↓ O_2 transport and uptake leading to a ↓ ability to hold one's breath	**Increased** Alkalosis causes an ↑ O_2 transport and uptake leading to a ↑ ability to hold one's breath
Urine pH	**Decreased** **Acidic urine-** kidneys compensate by excreting H+ in urine and retaining bicarbonate	**Increased** **Alkaline urine-** Kidneys compensate by retaining H+ and excreting bicarbonate in urine
Saliva pH	**Decreased** **Acidic saliva-** ↑ levels of CO_2 and carbonic acid due to hypoventilation	**Increased** **Alkaline saliva-** ↓ levels of CO_2 & carbonic acid due to hyperventilation

NOTES:

CAUSES OF METABOLIC ACIDOSIS AND ALKALOSIS

METABOLIC ACIDOSIS

1. **Inefficient formation of ATP-** an uncoupling of the Kreb's cycle from the oxidative phosphorylation system, caused by increasing oxidative stress, will lead to the creation and formation of organic acid metabolites in the cell

2. **The incomplete digestion/oxidation of proteins, fats and carbohydrates** due to diminished or depleted enzymes or stomach acid will lead to the build up of organic acids

3. **Increasing kidney stress.** Kidneys fail to process and eliminate H^+.

4. **Anaerobic respiration** causes a ↑ production of lactic and pyruvic acids due to general lack of oxygenation through poor breathing techniques.

5. **Renal loss** of bicarbonate, sodium and potassium

6. **Stress-** excess stimulation of the sympathetic nervous system creates increased cellular metabolism and concentrations of acidic metabolites

7. **A deficiency in vitamins and minerals** used as buffers by the body

8. **Lack of exercise**: body fails to clean and filter lymph

9. **Liver dysfunction** leads to failure of liver dependent urea cycle to flush out acids

10. **Heavy metals** and other oxidative catalysts

11. **Microbes-** bacteria, funguses etc. produce acidic waste

12. **Consumption of organic acids**: alcohol, sodas, coffee

13. **Drugs**: both prescription and recreational

14. **Severe diarrhea and deep vomiting**, which cause the loss of excess bicarbonate.

METABOLIC ALKALOSIS

1. **Use of diuretics-** Cause water, cation and chloride depletion, while bicarbonate is retained. Loss of H^+, K^+ and Mg^+ exceeds loss of sodium.

2. **Loss of acid-** loss of gastric fluid (Excessive vomiting), poor urinary retention of H^+

3. **Chloride depletion-** adrenal fatigue, loss of gastric juice, poor retention of Cl^-

4. **Excess secretion of aldosterone** from the adrenal cortex- Causes a large amount of sodium to be re-absorbed and urinary loss of H^+, Cl^- and K^+ ions

5. **Alkaline drugs-** e.g. the H_2 blockers of stomach acidity

6. **Excess consumption of bicarbonate-** Causes a decreased level of H^+; antacids

www.BloodChemistryAnalysis.com

NOTES:

CAUSES OF RESPIRATORY ACIDOSIS AND ALKALOSIS

RESPIRATORY ACIDOSIS

The cause of respiratory acidosis is **hypoventilation**, i.e. CO_2 is being blown off at a slower rate than it is being produced, which is usually caused by insufficient respirations or air exchange.

1. **Hypoventilation in compensation for metabolic alkalosis**

2. Acute respiratory acidosis can be seen in **asthma**

3. **High blood pressure**: As blood pressure increases, the aorta and carotid arteries carry more oxygenated blood past the chemoreceptors, which are stimulated and begin to lower the respiratory rate by changing rate and depth of breathing. This can lead to respiratory acidosis.

4. A mild respiratory acidosis occurs at night due to diminished respiration, which is one of the contributors to acidic urine first thing in the morning.

More emergency type situations:

5. **Head damage** can lead to damage of the respiratory center in the Medulla oblongata, which causes decreased respiration.

6. **Chest trauma** leading to compromised breathing rate and depth

7. **Respiratory diseases-** Chronic respiratory acidosis can be seen in respiratory diseases such as emphysema and pneumonia, which have an increase in dead air space in the lungs and a decreased pulmonary membrane surface area. This causes the lungs to not function normally. Acidosis develops slowly over a period of time.

8. **Obstruction to the respiratory passages**

RESPIRATORY ALKALOSIS

Respiratory alkalosis is often called stress or anxiety alkalosis because it can be caused by situations of extreme physiological stress. Too much acid is "blown off" from increased respirations or **hyperventilation**. Some of the causes include:

1. **Chronic and acute anxiety-** respiratory alkalosis is often called stress alkalosis

2. **Low blood pressure**, which causes a decreased flow of oxygenated blood through the aortic and carotid arteries, thus stimulating the respiratory centers to increase respiratory rate.

3. **Shock**

4. **Sepsis**

5. **Head trauma** may cause damage to the respiratory centers, which could lead to hyperventilation

6. **Psychoneurosis causing hyperventilation** and an excess loss of CO_2. In cases of hyperventilation of psychogenic origin, the increase in alkalosis causes the tingly sensation around the mouth and in the fingertips. Because of hyperventilation, blood is slowed to the brain so the respiratory center tells the body to increase respirations. In psychogenic hyperventilation, the symptoms of tingling and feeling of smothering continue to worsen.

7. **High altitudes** can cause a lowered concentration of oxygen, which triggers an increased respiration that lowers CO_2 concentration.

www.BloodChemistryAnalysis.com

NOTES:

COMMON SIGNS AND SYMPTOMS OF ACIDOSIS AND ALKALOSIS

ACIDOSIS	ALKALOSIS
• Anxiety	• Bad breath
• Diarrhea	• Cellulite
• Poor digestion and assimilation of food	• Constipation
• Dilated pupils	• Cold, clammy hands and feet
• Fatigue, especially in early morning	• Dizziness
• Headaches, occipital to frontal	• Fatigue in mornings, hard to arise from bed
• High blood pressure and rapid heart beat	• Headaches, side of head, temples (migraine)
• Hyperactivity	• Excitability of nervous system
• Insomnia	• Indigestion, fermentation
• Nervousness	• Introverted behavior, depression
• Restless legs	• Leg and muscle cramps, tetany
• Shortness of breath	• Low blood pressure
• Strong appetite	• Paleness
• Warm, dry hands and feet	• Slow pulse
• Dry mouth	• Sluggishness
• Allergies	• Poor digestion and assimilation of food due to decreased gastric secretion
• Poor retention of important mineral nutrients	• Joint and muscle pain
• Inefficient function of kidneys, lungs and adrenal glands	• Allergies- asthma
• Inflammation	• Poor retention of important mineral nutrients
• Skin irritations	
• Arthritis	

NOTES:

SECONDARY BUFFERING SYSTEMS

Alkaline minerals

- The body uses the acidic and alkaline properties of various minerals to help buffer the blood.

- When the blood becomes too acidic, the other fluids, especially the lymphatic fluid, will move into a less optimal acidic range by releasing alkaline minerals to buffer the blood and bring it back into an alkaline range.

- The family of mineral compounds that neutralize acids are the carbonic salts, symbolized as $AlkCO_3$ in the formula below.

- Alk stands for any of the 4 alkaline or basic elements: Sodium (Na^+) Calcium (Ca_2^+) Potassium (K^+) and Magnesium (Mg_2^+).

- When these carbonic salts meet with acids, the alkaline minerals making up the carbonic salts will combine with the acid to create a salt.

For example:

$$AlkCO_3 \quad + \quad H_2SO_4 \quad = \quad AlkSO_4 \quad + \quad H_2O \quad + \quad CO_2$$

| Carbonic salt | Sulfuric acid | Sulfuric salt | Water | Carbon dioxide |

This reaction has taken a strong acid and combined it with an alkaline salt to form a sulfuric salt, a compound easily excreted from the kidney without any harm.

The Liver and the Urea Cycle

The urea cycle of the liver combines carbon dioxide with ammonia (produced from the oxidation of the amino acid glutamine) and forms urea, which is excreted by the kidney.

The Digestive system

The following scenarios detail the digestive systems role in maintaining optimal pH:

NOTES:

a. **Acid blood:**

The digestive system helps buffer an acidic blood by supplying bicarbonate and other alkaline forming elements from the digestive enzyme systems of the small intestines to help buffer the acids.

Unfortunately this leaves a more acidic environment in the small intestine causing the liver and pancreatic secretions of digestive enzymes to not function optimally leading to digestion dysfunction.

b. **Alkaline blood:**

The digestive system helps buffer an alkaline blood by supplying acidic elements from the stomach in order to buffer the alkalinity.

This leaves a more alkaline environment in the stomach.

In this situation the digestion in the stomach becomes compromised and a state of hypochlorhydria exists.

Ammonia

A method that the body can use in short-term situations is the release of ammonia, which is very alkaline. This method is used when there are less than optimal amounts of alkaline minerals in the body fluids, or insufficient levels of minerals can be mustered in a short term situation.

Clinical assessment of 2° buffering systems

The best way to make a clinical assessment of the secondary buffering systems is to observe the buffering activity of the saliva in response to an acid challenge. This can be appreciated with Dr. Bieler's Salivary pH acid challenge test.

NOTES:

DR. BIELER'S SALIVARY PH ACID CHALLENGE

Background

Dr. Bieler's test is a dynamic measurement of the body's alkaline mineral reserves- one of the secondary buffering systems of the body. We are looking to see whether the body has the reserves necessary to respond to an acid challenge. During this test we challenge the body with acid in the form of lemon juice. The initial acidity of the lemon juice will cause the saliva to buffer this acidity over the course of a few minutes by becoming more alkaline. We expect the saliva to get more alkaline to show that the body can respond to an acid challenge by marshalling up the necessary alkaline mineral reserves. If there are enough alkaline minerals in the body, the body will use them as a buffer. If there is an alkaline mineral insufficiency, the body may start to use ammonia as a buffer, which is an indication of low mineral reserves.

This test also allows us to see how stress and sympathetic dominance impact minerals reserves in the body. Increasing levels of stress to the point of adrenal exhaustion will cause the loss of the primary mineral reserves, which are composed of the alkaline minerals potassium, magnesium, sodium and calcium. In ideal situations the kidneys use these alkaline reserves to buffer metabolic acids that come through the tubules. In times of mineral insufficiency and stress, the body will resort to using ammonia, which combines with acid and is secreted in the urine as ammonium salts. The ammonia buffering system is used in cases when there is a deficiency in the alkaline minerals. In these situations the urine may have a strong ammonia smell.

The buffering activity measured in this test occurs in the mouth, salivary ducts and saliva. It is a measure of short term buffering, using the secondary buffering systems and does not rely on stomach absorption of the lemon juice for its effect.

Discussion

The alkaline mineral reserves get taken up into the lymphatic fluid, where they are used as a buffer for extracellular acids.

- The saliva, as a measure of lymph fluid, is the ideal place to measure such activity.

- The mineral reserve buffer can be easily overwhelmed by increased levels of acidic metabolites, causing a progressively acidic lymphatic fluid and hence an acidic saliva.

NOTES:

Directions

1. Cut seven 2" strips of pH paper and lay out on paper towel

2. Prepare lemon juice drink: 1 tablespoon of lemon juice and 1 tablespoon of water

3. Have patient make a pool of saliva in mouth and dip half of the strip, remove and measure pH. Record as baseline

4. Have patient drink lemon juice, check pH and start timing

5. Test and record pH every minute for 5 minutes

When would you run this test?

- To check the alkaline mineral reserves in the body

- To see the impact that chronic stress has on these mineral reserves.

NOTES:

Normal patterns

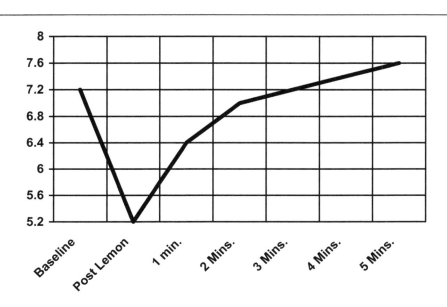

The initial salivary pH of 7.2 drops immediately after the acid challenge and takes a few minutes to climb up into the alkaline range. The slow climb up to 7.6 at 5 minutes indicates healthy mineral reserves

Base-line	Lemon	1 min.	2 mins	3 mins	4 mins	5 mins
7.2	5.2	6.4	7.0	7.2	7.4	7.6

NOTES:

Abnormal patterns seen in Dr. Bieler's salivary pH acid challenge test

1. The alkaline reaction

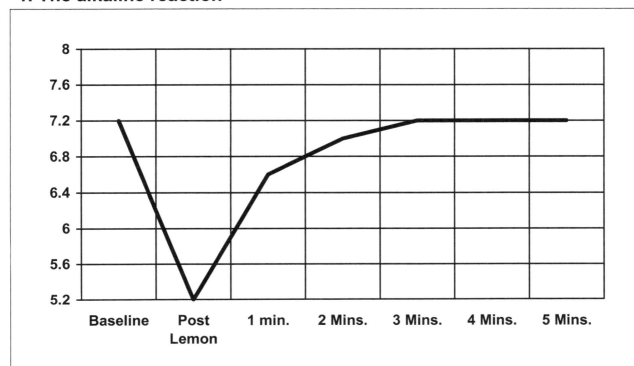

The alkaline reaction is a fairly normal reaction to a sudden increase of acid into the body but there are the beginnings of a tendency to drift towards mineral insufficiency. The Mineral reserves are intact but the buffering systems are not able to drive the pH as alkaline as the normal curve.

Base-line	Lemon	1 min.	2 mins	3 mins	4 mins	5 mins
7.2	5.2	6.6	7.0	7.2	7.2	7.2

NOTES:

2. Mineral insufficiency

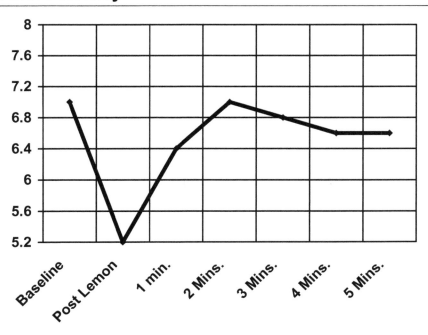

In the mineral insufficiency pattern the initial salivary pH of 7.2 drops immediately with the acid challenge and takes a few minutes to climb up to the alkaline range.

The slow climb up to a pH of 6.8 at 2 minutes starts to look like the normal curve, but it fails to completely alkalinize the saliva. This is an indication of mineral insufficiency. There are mineral reserves present but they are not replete enough to fully buffer the acidity.

The more the curve begins to drop the weaker the reserves are.

Base-line	Lemon	1 min.	2 mins	3 mins	4 mins	5 mins
7.0	5.2	6.4	7.0	6.8	6.6	6.6

NOTES:

3. Hypersympathetic overload with mineral insufficiency

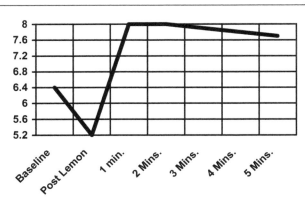

Notice that the starting point is acidic to begin with at 6.4. This pattern is already displaying signs of buffering problems before the test has started. The alkaline spike after 1 minute indicates that ammonia is being used as a buffer. Ammonia, and not minerals, is being released. The patient may notice the ammonia response in the urine, which may have an ammonia smell.

This patient will complain of being wiped out and fatigued. They probably do not sleep well, are stressed and complain of feeling depleted. Any types of stress reduction techniques are essential for these people along with adrenal restoration. They often complain of not being able to relax. Notice also that the curve does not come down very quickly. The ammonia is quite a long term buffer.

Base-line	Lemon	1 min.	2 mins	3 mins	4 mins	5 mins
6.4	5.2	8	8	7.9	7.8	7.7

NOTES:

4. Hypersympathetic overload with signs of mineral sufficiency

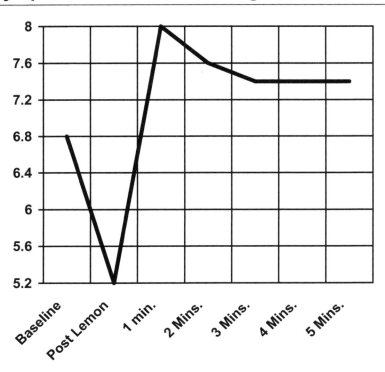

This curve looks similar to the curve above in the hyper sympathetic patient. There is still the ammonia spike but after 2 minutes there is signs of mineral reserve activity coming online because the pH is beginning to drop into the normal range.

Base-line	Lemon	1 min.	2 mins	3 mins	4 mins	5 mins
6.8	5.2	8.0	7.6	7.4	7.4	7.4

NOTES:

5. Loss of alkaline reserves

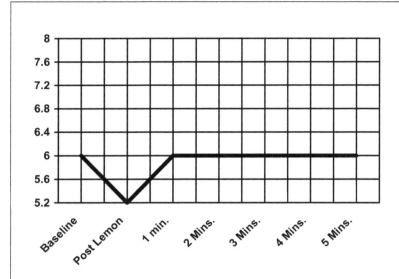

This pattern is an indication of a loss of buffering capacity, at least in the short term.

There is probably cell rigidity and the kidneys are probably no longer reclaiming acidity. The first morning urine pH may be alkaline. Check the urine dipstick for any abnormalities and run a blood chemistry screen and CBC.

Base-line	Lemon	1 min.	2 mins	3 mins	4 mins	5 mins
6.0	5.2	6.0	6.0	6.0	6.0	6.0

<u>Related Tests</u>

- Urinary adrenal stress test

- Oxidata free radical test

- Urine pH

- Saliva pH

- Breath holding time

- Respiration rate

NOTES:

Dr. Bieler's Salivary pH Acid Challenge Handout

Name:_____   Date:_____

Dr. Bieler's test is a dynamic measurement of your body's alkaline mineral reserves, which are one of the systems that your body uses to deal with acid and alkaline imbalances. We are looking to see whether your body has the reserves necessary to respond to an acid challenge. During this test you will challenge your body with acid in the form of lemon juice. The initial acidity of the lemon juice will cause the saliva to buffer the acidity of the lemon juice over the course of a few minutes by becoming more alkaline. We expect the saliva to get more alkaline to show that the body can respond to an acid challenge by marshalling up the necessary alkaline minerals.
This test also allows us to see how stress and sympathetic dominance impact minerals reserves in your body. Increasing levels of stress can the loss of these primary mineral reserves.

Instructions

1. You will be given a roll of pH paper to do this test, which will take about 7 minutes to complete and consists of taking the pH of your saliva 7 times
2. Cut seven 2" strips of pH paper and lay them out on paper towel
3. Prepare your lemon juice drink: 1 tbls of lemon juice and 1 tbls of water
4. To take a saliva pH reading: Make a pool of saliva in your mouth and dip half of the strip into this pool of saliva, remove and measure pH on the chart that comes with the pH paper. Do not put the whole strip in your mouth or hold it in for too long.
5. Record this first reading as a baseline on the chart below
6. Drink the lemon drink, check your pH again and start timing
7. Test and record your saliva pH every minute on for 5 minutes
8. Record all your results on the form below

Chart for recording your results

Date of test:

Baseline	Lemon	1 minute	2 minutes	3 minutes	4 minutes	5 minutes

Oxidative
Stress

NOTES:

OXIDATIVE STRESS

What is oxidative stress?

Oxidative stress is a disturbance in the balance between the reactive oxygen species or free radicals and the antioxidant levels in the favor of the reactive oxygen species.

What are Free radicals?

- Free radicals are extremely reactive and unstable molecules that contain unpaired electrons.

- Most molecules have their electron orbitals occupied by paired electrons of opposite spin, which is a state that is both more energetically favorable and more stable.

- The unpaired electron in the outer shell is responsible for the instability and reactivity of all free radicals.

- Once they have been created they tend to spread and multiply by chain reactions with other, less reactive molecules.

- These chain reactions cause most of the cellular damage of free radicals and can only be stopped by antioxidants, which have the ability to donate an electron and thus neutralize the problem.

- It should be remembered that free radicals are also a by-product of normal metabolism and pro-oxidative reactions are a part of normal physiological activity that are used to neutralize toxins etc.

- They become harmful if they are not immediately neutralized.

How are free radicals created in the body?

Free radicals are formed either endogenously or from exposure to exogenous toxins.

Some of the endogenous causes of free radicals include:

- The mitochondria, which is one of the major sources of endogenous free radicals formed by the enzymatically controlled transfer of energized electrons for ATP generation in Oxidative phosphorylation

- The liver, which creates free radicals as part of the cytochrome P450 system of detoxification

NOTES:

- The Immune system, which uses oxidative species such as hypochlorite to neutralize microbes and their waste products

- The Immune, endocrine and neurological systems, which respond to excessive stress via neurotransmitter activity that produces free radicals

Some of the exogenous causes of free radicals include:

1. The primary contribution to increased free radicals is the exposure to xenobiotics, which not only causes the liver and adrenal cortex to produce free radicals but also depletes specific cellular antioxidants such as glutathione, vitamin C or vitamin E. Some of the common xenobiotics we are exposed to include

- Pesticides and Herbicides

- Food additives

- Household chemicals and Industrial solvents

- Fuels and Fuel additives

- Fertilizers

- Drugs

- Air pollution

- Alcohol

2. Exposure to excess ultraviolet light

3. Exposure to radiation

4. Exposure to trauma

5. Exposure to cold

What are the effects of free radicals and oxidative stress in the body?

Free radical or oxidative stress is thought to be a major factor in many chronic illnesses. Free radicals have been associated with the following:

- Diabetes and potentially the destruction of pancreatic beta cells, which is a leading cause of type 1 diabetes

NOTES:

- Tissue damage to colonic mucosal cells in ulcerative colitis and Inflammatory Bowel Disease

- Increased risk of breast and cervical cancer from the increased levels of lipid peroxides, which are oxidized fats, in the tissue

- Damage to cell membranes, which causes impaired cellular transport, cell-to-cell communication and binding

- Damage to liver cells

- Disordered calcium, magnesium and potassium cellular movement

- Interference in oxidative phosphorylation and the ability to convert the bi-products of the Kreb's cycle into ATP

- Oxidation of LDL, an increased risk of cardiovascular disease

- Cataract formation

- Decreased energy production, a major cause of chronic fatigue

- Depressed immune function

- Alterations in the nucleic acids that make up the DNA, leading to increased cancer formation

- Rheumatoid arthritis, systemic lupus Erythematosus and glomerular diseases, which have been shown to have increased levels of free radicals and lipid peroxides

- Systemic and local inflammation

In-office tests for Oxidative Stress

- While the significance of free radicals and oxidative stress has been known for years, until now it has been difficult to assess for oxidative stress in the office.

- Functional Terrain Analysis utilizes the Oxidata free radical test to evaluate both oxidative stress status and antioxidant reserves.

- This test is a "gateway" test that should be run to see if it is necessary to order the more expensive and elaborate acetaminophen/salicylate challenge tests and liver detoxification panels.

NOTES:

OXIDATA FREE RADICAL TEST

Background

- Free radicals are molecules that contain unpaired electrons. Unpaired electrons are by-products of normal metabolism and xenobiotics reactions.

- These molecules are very unstable and reactive with other molecules.

- Once free radical reactions begin, they tend to multiply by chain reactions with cellular material.

- The chain reactions tend to have long lasting effects and the potential to cause cellular damage (i.e. cell membrane or DNA disruption). Free radical or oxidative stress is thought to be a major factor in many chronic illnesses.

- High levels of free radicals are associated with exposure to environmental pollutants, inflammatory diseases and low antioxidant status.

- It is important to remember that our body needs a certain amount of oxidative stress to deal with toxins, microbes etc. Both too much and too little oxidative stress is a problem.

Antioxidants

- Antioxidants, such as vitamins A,C, and E, lipoic acid and glutathione, are thought to stop free radicals and protect the body from cellular damage.

- Antioxidants both treat and prevent further oxidative damage.

Discussion

The Oxidata Free Radical Test determines the presence of free radical or oxidative stress and, by association, antioxidant status.

- The test measures the distal end of the polyunsaturated fat chain where aldehyde forms from free radical reaction.

- Aldehydes, present in many body compartments (serum, blood etc.) are found in highest levels in urine.

- Urine aldehyde measurement is reportedly 50 times more sensitive than blood aldehyde levels.

NOTES:

When would you run this test?

1. To help identify oxidative stress patterns in the body
2. To assess antioxidant status

Directions

Ask patients to stop all supplements two days prior to test. It is best to collect the first morning urine and refrigerate specimen in an airtight container if they have a later appointment.

- Draw urine into the dropper supplied with the test kit

- Break open the top of the glass ampoule, which contains the reagent

- Place urine into the ampoule

- Wait five minutes, then interpret the color change from the chart and record result

Results

Pink color or +1	**Optimal reading indicating optimum oxidation, healthy and normal**
Clear or 0	**Abnormally reduced oxidation and low electron potential**
Red +2	**Moderate oxidation- level of free radical activity and oxidative stress is beginning to Increase**
Dark red +3	**Heavy oxidation- levels of free radicals and oxidative stress are too high**

NOTES:

Clinical implications

LOW- Clear or 0

Clinical Implication	Additional information
Loss of high energy electrons	A low redox is associated with the loss of high-energy electrons in the urine causing a low electron potential. Electrons, produced from glycolosis and the Kreb's cycle, are not being used by the cell's mitochondria, because of mitochondrial membrane problems. This leads to an inability to produce ATP and increasing levels of fatigue. The electrons are excreted in the urine. This situation has been called Ox-phos derailment i.e. the oxidative phosphorylation process has been derailed from the Kreb's cycle. This may be due to mitochondrial membrane dysfunction or a lack of ubiquinone or CoQ10, the last enzyme in the oxidative phosphorylation process, which "pulls" the high energy intermediates through the enzymatic pathway.
Degenerative diseases **Premature tissue Aging**	An increased loss of high energy electrons is associated with degenerative diseases and premature tissue aging

NOTES:

HIGH- INCREASING OXIDATIVE STRESS

+2 or Red color change

Clinical Implication	Additional information
Liver stress	The liver uses oxidation to perform some of its functions. Increasing oxidative stress only puts more strain on the liver
Kidney stress	The glomerulus of the kidney is very sensitive to oxidative damage. Many of the xenotoxins that contribute to oxidative stress can damage the kidneys and block glomerular function
Pancreas stress- GI and blood sugar dysregulation	Increased oxidation will put stress on the pancreas, which will impact its function leading to blood sugar problems and maldigestion
Adrenal stress	Increased oxidation is one of the adrenal stressors.
Lymphatic congestion	Increasing lymphatic congestion can lead to increasing levels of oxidative stress as the body cannot clean and filter waste
Fatigue	There is a likelihood of a decreased production of high-energy electron intermediates from the Kreb's cycle, which affects the cells ability to produce energy. As oxidation increases there is a reduced output of ATP from the mitochondria, which leads to fatigue. This process has been called a Kreb's cycle or Tri Carboxylic Acid (TCA) disruption.

NOTES:

+3 or Dark Red color change

Clinical Implications	Additional Information
Lymphatic stress	The lymph system becomes overburdened with the presence of pro-oxidative toxins that cause increased oxidative stress
Xenotoxins	An increased likelihood of the possible presence of xenotoxins in the body, which is increasing the oxidative stress
Greatly reduced ATP production	High oxidative stress causes less and less production of high-energy electron intermediates from the Kreb's cycle's, which affects the cells ability to produce energy. As oxidation increases there is a greatly reduced output of ATP from the mitochondria, which leads to fatigue and a slowing down of essential enzymatic pathways. This process has been called a Kreb's cycle or Tri Carboxylic Acid (TCA) disruption.
Maldigestion	The effect of increasing oxidative stress on the pancreas can impact digestive enzyme production leading to maldigestion
Blood sugar dysregulation	The effect of increasing oxidative stress on the pancreas can impact the release of insulin from the beta islet cells.

NOTES:

URINE VITAMIN C TEST

Discussion

 Optimal levels of vitamin C are needed to maintain healthy connective tissue, adrenal glands, red blood cells and capillary walls.

- Vitamin C is a threshold substance, meaning it is not excreted until the ascorbic acid level in the blood exceeds a certain value related to the degree of tissue saturation.

- When vitamin C in the serum reaches approximately 1.2 mg/dl, the kidneys stop reabsorbing it.

- Vitamin C is stored in many tissues of the body, most notably in the kidneys, adrenals and lungs.

- If vitamin C intake is too high, the intestines fail to absorb it and it is eliminated through the feces.

- If vitamin C reserves in the body are low, then little will be excreted in the urine. It takes more drops of urine to decolorize the reagent indicating less vitamin C in each drop of urine.

- This test measures the ascorbic acid, which is the antioxidant portion of the vitamin C complex. People taking the ascorbate form of vitamin C may appear deficient in this test.

Normal values

1-5 drops of urine will decolorize the reagent

When would you run this test?

1. To assess absorption, utilization and tissue storage of vitamin C

2. As part of the functional urinalysis panel

NOTES:

Clinical implications

HIGH (>5 drops of urine to decolorize reagent)

Clinical Implication	Additional information
Dietary insufficiency or deficiency of vitamin C	Very common in people who eat refined foods, women during pregnancy and lactation, children, immune suppressed people and people with many diseases.

Low vitamin C is associated with the following

- Adrenal insufficiency, exhaustion and fatigue

- ↑ capillary permeability: bruising, bleeding gums, gum disorders

- Joint pain, aching joints, loss of bone mass and stiffness

- Lowered resistance to infections, sore throat, laryngitis, and tonsillitis

- Slow healing of wounds and fractures

- Impaired digestion,

- Shortness of breath,

- Scurvy

- Tissue and collagen disorders

Interfering Factors

Many people taking large doses of vitamin C in the form of ascorbates may show severe vitamin c deficiency in this test.

Related tests

- Oxidata Free Radical Test

Patterns Between In-Office Tests

NOTES:

Functional Terrain Analysis Patterns

Introduction

This section focuses on the patterns or combinations that exist between 2 or more elements and the diagnostic information that can be found with such an analysis.

When analyzing the patterns it might be useful to look back at each of the individual component.

The following is a glossary of terms that are used in describing some of these patterns:

Digestion: The breakdown of food particles in the GI tract

Absorption: Passage of food particles across the intestinal mucosa

Assimilation: Nutrients are assimilated into the blood stream

Utilization: Passage of nutrients from the blood through the cell membrane

NOTES:

Patterns

- Assimilation and digestion

- Acid/Alkaline Assessment

- Electrolyte assessment

- Calcium and mineralization

- Macronutrient Maldigestion Patterns

- Urine bilirubin with urine urobilinogen levels

NOTES:

Assimilation and digestion

PATTERN	INTERPRETATION	CLINICAL IMPLICATIONS
↑ Indican ↑ Sediment	Hypochlorhydria Pancreatic Insufficiency Leaky Gut Syndrome	• High indican levels are a reflection of protein mal-digestion and an excess of undigested food particles. Both of these are signs of hypochlorhydria. • High sediment reflects poor breakdown of the absorbed nutrients due to leaky gut syndrome or pancreatic insufficiency (lack or decreased activity of digestive enzymes). Patients with this pattern may inform you that their appetite is extremely high and that they eat even when they are not hungry.
↑ Indican → Sediment	Maldigestion Malabsorption	This pattern indicates poor digestion and absorption of nutrients across the gut wall into the blood and cell. There may be damage to the small intestine mucosa, as a result of a bacterial overgrowth or other infection, causing decreased permeability or a reduced intestinal mucosal surface area. One of the symptoms of this might be an excessive appetite. The maldigestion may be from hypochlorhydria or pancreatic insufficiency.
N indican → Sediment	Malabsorption Deficient Dietary intake	This pattern indicates malabsorption without maldigestion. There may also be a relatively deficient dietary intake as a result of poor diet or a relative reduction in food intake. There may be damage to the small intestine mucosa.
N indican ↑ Sediment	Leaky Gut Syndrome Vitamin/mineral deficiencies	This pattern indicates good digestion but an increased permeability. With increased sediment there is evidence of abnormal metabolites being absorbed through a leaky gut. The increase in abnormal metabolites may be due to a deficiency in minerals and vitamins that act as co-enzymes to the enzymatic processes of digestion. This is a pattern often seen in people who are eating large amounts of one food group

www.BloodChemistryAnalysis.com

NOTES:

PATTERN	INTERPRETATION	CLINICAL IMPLICATIONS
↑ Indican ↑ Calcium	Hypochlorhydria	This pattern is associated with poor digestion, especially proteins, due to an inability to produce enough acidity in the stomach i.e. Hypochlorhydria. Since half of the circulating calcium is bound to protein, a protein deficiency resulting from an HCL deficiency could increase the ionized (diffusible) calcium, which is readily excreted in the urine.
↑ Indican ↓ Calcium	Lowered systemic pH Bicarbonate deficiency ↑ Phosphorous loss	This pattern may suggest a high loss of phosphorous due to increased systemic acidity. This may be result from a deficiency in bicarbonate buffers. There is decreased calcium because it is being used to buffer excess hydrogen ions in the extracellular fluid.

www.BloodChemistryAnalysis.com

NOTES:

Acid/Alkaline Assessment

PATTERN	INTERPRETATION	CLINICAL IMPLICATIONS
↑ Resp. rate → Breath hold → Urine pH ↑ Saliva pH	**Metabolic Acidosis**	1. Alkaline saliva- the respiratory system kicks in by increasing the rate and depth of breathing to blow off as much CO2 as possible. This will lower the carbonic acid levels in the body leading to alkaline saliva. 2. Acidic urine- this represents the kidney excreting H+ 3. Increased respiratory rate- The body is attempting to blow off CO2 to decrease carbonic acid levels 4. Decreased breath holding time- acidosis causes a decreased oxygen transport and uptake, thus leading to a decreased ability to hold ones breath
↑/↓ Resp. rate → Breath hold ↓ Urine pH → Saliva pH	**Respiratory Acidosis**	1. Acid saliva- due to the increased levels of CO2 and carbonic acid 2. Acidic urine- due to the kidney excretion of H+ 3. Increased respiratory rate- The body is attempting to blow off CO2 to decrease carbonic acid levels that have built up as a result of the hypoventilation, which is a hallmark of respiratory acidosis 4. Decreased breath holding time- acidosis causes a decreased oxygen transport and uptake, thus leading to a decreased ability to hold ones breath

www.BloodChemistryAnalysis.com

NOTES:

PATTERN	INTERPRETATION	CLINICAL IMPLICATIONS
↑/↓ Resp. rate ↑ Breath hold ↑ Urine pH ↑ Saliva pH	**Respiratory Alkalosis** **(Also known as stress or anxiety alkalosis)**	1. Alkaline saliva- due to the increased loss of CO2 and carbonic acid 2. Alkaline urine- due to the kidney retention of H+ 3. The respiratory rate may be increased or decreased- The body is attempting to blow off CO2 to decrease carbonic acid levels but the respiration patterns are often irregular 4. Increased breath holding time- alkalosis causes an increased oxygen transport and uptake, thus leading to an increased ability to hold ones breath
↓ Resp. rate ↑ Breath hold ↑ Urine pH ↓ Saliva pH	**Metabolic alkalosis**	1. Acidic saliva- a slowing of the respiration rate will cause more carbonic acid in the extracellular fluids leading to an acidic saliva 2. Alkaline urine- due to kidney excretion of bicarbonate and retention H+ 3. Decreased respiratory rate- due to the suppression of the respiratory centers (the body is attempting to lessen the blow off CO2 to increase carbonic acid levels) 4. Increased breath holding time- alkalosis causes an increased oxygen transport and uptake, thus leading to an increased ability to hold ones breath

NOTES:

Electrolyte assessment

PATTERN	INTERPRETATION	CLINICAL IMPLICATIONS
→ Urine chloride ← Urine pH	**Excess alkaline reserves**	The extracellular fluid is alkaline. Large amounts of chloride are reabsorbed resulting in a decreased urine chloride. The renal tubules release bicarbonate and hold onto H+ in order to buffer the excess alkalinity. The urine becomes alkaline. This is a normal variation.
← Urine chloride → Urine pH	**Excess acid reserves** **Electrolyte insufficiency**	The extracellular fluid is acidic. The body copes by causing the renal tubules to reabsorb bicarbonate in order to buffer the acidity. Urine becomes more acidic. Chloride ion reabsorption is decreased resulting in a high urine chloride . This is a normal variation.
→ Urine chloride → Urine pH	**Potassium deficiency** **Salt deficiency**	The blood is deficient in potassium, from eating the standard American diet, too much refined sugar or diuretic use, produces this pattern. The body is excreting H+ and retaining chloride, which leads to an acidic urine. Because of the low pH the body excretes more potassium. If patient has this pattern and reports that their urine output is low consider sodium deficiency because the body is retaining chloride and excreting H+.
← Urine chloride ← Urine pH ← Calcium	**Excess salt**	In this pattern the body is excreting bicarbonate and chloride as well as calcium. This pattern is seen in people who consume excess amounts of salt.

155

www.BloodChemistryAnalysis.com

NOTES:

PATTERN	INTERPRETATION	CLINICAL IMPLICATIONS
↑ Urine chloride ↑ Urine pH → Calcium	**Excess potassium**	This pattern is similar but different from the one above. In this pattern the body is excreting bicarbonate and chloride, but retaining calcium. This pattern is seen in salt deficient diets or people who are taking too much potassium.

NOTES:

Calcium and mineralization

PATTERN	INTERPRETATION	CLINICAL IMPLICATIONS
↘ Urine pH ↘ Calcium	**Excess stomach acid**	Excess stomach acid- possible causes often associated with this pattern are: • Very high protein diet • Magnesium deficiency, because magnesium neutralizes HCl in the stomach. • Medications • Taking Betaine HCl • Acid retention due to kidney disease • Ketosis from fasting or diabetes
↘Urine pH ↖ Calcium	**Complex carbohydrate deficiency** **Alkaline mineral deficiency**	Complex carbohydrate deficiency associated with the standard American Diet i.e. fast food diet high in sugar and protein (↑ sugar can cause ↑ calcium in the urine) Alkaline minerals are being depleted in order to alkalinize the cell. A pattern seen in respiratory acidosis and respiratory conditions such as asthma and emphysema and after an acute asthma attack.
↖ Urine pH ↘ Calcium	**Hypochlorhydria**	Hypochlorhydria can cause poor protein digestion leading to low calcium levels since half of the calcium is bound to protein. It is also suggestive of the following: • Poor protein and calcium digestion and transportation due to • Hypochlorhydria • Poor reserve levels of calcium in the bones • Fatty acid deficiency.

157

www.BloodChemistryAnalysis.com

NOTES:

PATTERN	INTERPRETATION	CLINICAL IMPLICATIONS
↑ Urine pH ↑ Calcium	**Protein deficiency**	This pattern can be due to protein deficiency due to low protein diet or poor protein absorption. Use of protease to increase absorption may be useful. The increase in calcium may be due to the intake of a non-ionizing form of calcium
N Urine pH ↓ Calcium	**Low calcium levels in body**	May be caused by insufficient intake of calcium or other factors that affect calcium digestion, absorption and utilization. Most of the unabsorbed calcium will be excreted in the stool.

NOTES:

Macronutrient Maldigestion Patterns

PATTERN	INTERPRETATION	CLINICAL IMPLICATIONS
→ Urine chloride ← S.G.	**Protein maldigestion**	This pattern indicates a difficulty in digesting protein either from a deficiency in protease enzyme or hypochlorhydria. This is associated with a loss of muscle mass, poor recovery time after exercise, hypoglycemia/blood sugar dysregulation, and poor utilization of calcium and magnesium, which must bind with amino acids to be fully assimilated. People with this pattern may also have intestinal mucosal integrity problems causing ileocecal valve problems, constipation and other lower bowel problems. This may be due to glutamine deficiencies.
→ Urine chloride → S.G.	**Fat maldigestion**	This pattern indicates a difficulty in dealing with fats either from a deficiency in lipase enzymes or poor bile emulsification. Your patients may talk about having a fat intolerance. This is associated with a deficiency in essential fatty acids, fat soluble nutrient deficiencies and liver and/or gallbladder problems.
← Urine chloride ← S.G.	**Fiber and carbohydrate maldigestion**	This pattern indicates fiber and carbohydrate maldigestion and metabolism, which may result from a deficiency in amylase or cellulase, or a high carbohydrate, low protein, low sodium and low fat diet. This pattern is associated with irritable bowel like symptoms, such as diarrhea. With this combination the pituitary increases the stimulation of ADH and GH to retain electrolytes. The patient may suffer from poor circulation, cold hands and feet, and a low sex drive.
← Urine chloride → S.G.	**Sugar maldigestion**	This pattern is common in people who have problem digesting and handling sugar. Patients may consume large amounts of carbohydrates and say that they are sugar intolerant. This pattern is associated with the following conditions: • Sugar handling difficulties • Malabsorption • Decreased cell permeability Sugar intolerance may also lead to depression, insomnia, emotional instability, and panic attacks.

NOTES:

Urine bilirubin with urine urobilinogen levels

PATTERN	INTERPRETATION	CLINICAL IMPLICATIONS
↑ bilirubin ↑ Urobilinogen	Liver dysfunction	This pattern has its origin in the liver with possible hepatocellular dysfunction or partial obstruction
↑ Bilirubin N Urobilinogen	Biliary Stasis	This pattern is associated with more of a gallbladder origin either biliary stasis with congested bile or gall stones
Neg Bilirubin ↑ Urobilinogen	Hemolytic in origin	This pattern is more hemolytic in origin. There is an increase in red blood cell destruction due to hemolytic anemia, oxidative stress, ↑ xenotoxins.

Other patterns:

Increased Oxidative Stress	↑ Oxidata test ↑ Urinary urobilinogen ↑ Hemolysed blood in urine

160

www.BloodChemistryAnalysis.com

NOTES:

Conditions and Functional Terrain Analysis Tests

CONDITION	HIGH	LOW
Adrenal hyperfunctioning		↓ Urine chloride
Adrenal hypofunctioning	↑ Urine chloride	
Alkaline mineral insufficiency	↑ Saliva pH ↑ Calcium oxalate sediment ↑ Urine chloride	↓ Saliva pH
Antioxidant insufficiency	↑ Oxidata test	
Bowel toxemia	↑ Indican	
Carbohydrate maldigestion	↑ Calcium phos. sediment ↑ Urine chloride ↑ Specific gravity ↑ Urine ketones	↓ Urine pH ↓ Saliva pH
Complex carbohydrate deficiency	↑ Urine Calcium	↓ Urine pH
Deficient dietary intake	Normal Indican	↓ Total sediment
Dysbiosis	↑ Indican	
Electrolyte insufficiency	↑ Urine chloride	↓ Urine pH
Electrolyte stress	↑ Urine pH	↓ Urine chloride

NOTES:

CONDITION	HIGH	LOW
Essential fatty acid deficiency		↓ Saliva pH
Excess protein intake	↑ Indican ↑ Uric acid sediment ↑ Urine ketones	↓ Urine calcium ↓ Urine pH
Excess stomach acidity		↓ Urine pH ↓ Calcium
Fat maldigestion	↑ Indican ↑ Calcium oxalate sediment	↓ Urine pH ↓ Saliva pH ↓ Urine chloride ↓ Specific gravity
Gallbladder insufficiency	↑ Calcium oxalate sediment ↑ Urine Bilirubin	
Hypochlorhydria	↑ Saliva pH ↑ Indican ↑ Uric acid sediment ↑ Urine chloride ↑ Urine pH	↓ Urine calcium
Hypothyroidism, Subclinical		↓ Basal body temp ↓ Iodine ↓ Achilles return reflex

NOTES:

CONDITION	HIGH	LOW
Immune dysfunction	↑ Urine pH	
Iodine insufficiency		↓ Iodine
Kidney stress	↑ 1st AM Urine pH ↑ Urine chloride ↑ Oxidata test	
Leaky gut syndrome	↑ Total sediment ↑ Indican	
Liver stress	↑ 1st AM Urine pH ↑ Urine bilirubin ↑ Urine ketones ↑ Urine urobilinogen	
Low calcium levels		↓ Urine calcium
Low redox potential		↓ Oxidata test
Malabsorption	↑ Indican	↓ Saliva pH ↓ Total urine sediment ↓ Urine chloride
Maldigestion	↑ Saliva pH ↑ Indican ↑ Oxidata test	↓ Urine pH ↓ Total sediment

NOTES:

CONDITION	HIGH	LOW
Metabolic acidosis	↑ Respiration rate ↑ Saliva pH	↓ Breath holding time ↓ Urine pH ↓ Calcium
Metabolic alkalosis	↑ Breath holding time ↑ Urine pH ↑ Calcium	↓ Respiration rate ↓ Saliva pH
Oxidative stress	↑ Oxidata test ↑ Urine chloride ↑ Urine bilirubin ↑ Urine urobilinogen ↑ Urine blood- hemolysed	↓ Lingual ascorbic acid
Pancreatic insufficiency	↑ Total sediment	↓ Urine pH ↓ Saliva pH
Protein deficiency	↑ Urine pH ↑ Urine calcium	

NOTES:

CONDITION	HIGH	LOW
Protein maldigestion	↑ Urine pH ↑ Indican ↑ Uric acid sediment ↑ Specific gravity ↑ Urine bilirubin	↓ Urine chloride
Respiratory acidosis	↑ Respiration rate ↑ Urine calcium	↓ Respiration rate ↓ Breath holding time ↓ Urine pH ↓ Saliva pH
Respiratory alkalosis	↑ Respiration rate ↑ Breath holding time ↑ Saliva pH ↑ Urine pH	↓ Respiration rate ↓ calcium

Forms and Handouts
for In-Office Testing

NOTES:

Patterns Chart for In-Office Lab Testing

Client's Name:_____ Practitioner:_____ Date:_____

Assimilation and Digestion Assessment

Test		Result		Interpretation:
Urine Indican Test	(0)			
Urine Sediment	(0.5)			
Urine Calcium	(Normal)			

↑ Indican ↑ Sediment	↑ Indican ↕ Sediment	N Indican ↓ Sediment	N Indican ↑ Sediment	↑ Indican ↑ Calcium	↑ Indican ↕ Calcium
Hypochlorhydria Panc. Insuff. Leaky Gut	Maldigestion Malabsorption	Malabsorption Deficient dietary intake	Leaky Gut Syndrome	Hypochlorhydria	↓ systemic pH Bicarbonate def. ↑ Phosph. loss

Acid/Alkaline Assessment: Respiration or Breath hold plus Urine pH, Saliva pH

Test		Result	Resp. Acid.	Met. Acid.	Resp. Alk.	Met. Alk.	Interpretation:
Resp Rate	(14-18)		> 19 or < 13	> 19	> 19 or < 13	< 13	
Breath Hold	(40-65)		< 40	< 40	>65	> 65	
Urine pH	(6.4-6.8)		< 6.4	<6.4	>6.8	>6.8	
Salivary pH	(7.1-7.4)		< 7.1	>7.4	>7.4	<7.1	

Electrolyte Assessment

Test		Result	Interpretation:
Urine Chloride (6 - 12)			
Urine ph	(6.4-6.8)		
Urine Calcium	(Normal)		

↑ Urine Chloride, ↑ Urine pH	↑ Urine Chloride, ↕ Urine pH	↓ Urine Chloride ↓ Urine pH	↑ Urine Chloride, ↑ Urine pH ↑ Calcium	↑ Urine Chloride, ↑ Urine pH ↓ Calcium
Excess alkaline reserves	Electrolyte Insufficiency	Potassium def.	Excess salt	Excess potassium

Calcium and Mineralization

Test		Result	Interpretation:
Urine pH	(6.4-6.8)		
Urine Calcium	(Normal)		

↑ Urine pH ↑ Urine calcium	↓ Urine pH ↑ Urine calcium	↑ Urine pH ↓ Urine calcium	↑ Urine pH ↑ Urine calcium	N Urine pH ↓ Urine calcium
Hypoglycemia ↑ Stomach acid Magnesium def.	Complex CHO Def. Alkaline mineral Def.	Hypochlorhydria	Protein deficiency	Low calcium

Macronutrient maldigestion patterns

Test		Result	Interpretation:
Urine Chloride	(6 – 12)		
Urine Specific Gravity	(1.015)		

↓ Urine Chloride, ↑ S.G.	↓ Urine Chloride, ↓ S.G.	↑ Urine Chloride, ↑ S.G.	↑ Urine Chloride, ↓ S.G.
Protein maldigestion	Fat maldigestion	Fiber/CHO Maldigestion Adrenal insufficiency	Sugar maldigestion

NOTES:

Results Form for In-Office Lab Testing

Client's Name:_____ Practitioner:_____

. Breath Hold (40-65)		2. Resp. Rate (14-18)		3. Salivary pH (7.1-7.4)		4. Urine pH (6.4-6.8)		
Date	Score	Date	Score	Date	Static pH	Date	1	2

. Dr. Bieler's Salivary pH Acid Challenge

Date	Baseline pH	Lemon	1 minute	2 minutes	3 minutes	4 minutes	5 minutes

. Zinc Taste Test

Date	Strength of taste	Seconds to taste	Result

Strength of Taste

Time (in Seconds)	1	2	3	4
1	Optimal			
2	Optimal			
3				
4		Mild		
5		Mild		
6				
7				
8			Moderate	
9			Moderate	
10				
11				
12				
13				
14			Severe	
15			Severe	

Optimal	Mild	Moderate	Severe
Immediate taste Strong Metallic	Not so strong taste Delayed metallic	No taste noted initially. Sweet or bitter	Tasteless or "tastes like water"

7. Dr. Kane's Mineral Assessment Test

Date		
Potassium Phosphate		
Zinc Sulfate		
Magnesium Chloride		
Copper Sulfate		
Potassium Chloride		
Potassium permanganate		
Ammonium molybdate		
1-3 Need to take	**4** Normal	**5-7** No need to take

NOTES:

. Urine S.G. (1.015)	
ate	Score

9. Achilles reflex

Date	Score

10. Urine Vitamin C Test

Date	Score

1. Urinary Chloride

Date	Score

1-5 ↓ Urinary chloride Adrenal Stress	6 - 12 Normal	>12 ↑ Urinary Chloride Adrenal Fatigue

12. Bowel toxicity Test/Urinary Indican

Date	Score

0 Normal	1-3 Mild Dysbiosis	4-7 Mod.	> 7 Severe Dysbiosis

3. Urine Calcium Test

Date	Score

Calcium Clear Light Turbidity	Normal Some Turbidity	↑ Calcium Heavy Turbidity Milky

14. Urine Sediment Test

Date	Total	Calc. Phos	Uric Acid	Calc. Ox.

Normal 0.5 ml Total Sediment	↑ **Calc. Phos** = Carbohydrate sediment ↑ **Uric acid** = Protein sediment ↑ **Calc. Oxalate** = Fat Sediment

5. Oxidata Free Radical Test

Date	Score

0 Low Oxidation	+1 Normal	+2 Moderate Oxidation	+3 High Oxidation

16. Iodine Patch Test

Date	Score

Color Lasts > 24 Hours Sufficient Iodine	Color fades < 24 hours Insufficient Iodine

7. Raglands Postural Hypotension Test

Date	Supine BP	Standing BP

1 Normal 6-10 point rise in systolic ressure	2 Fair Systolic pressure remains the same	3 Poor Up to 10 point drop in systolic pressure	4 Worse Up to 20 point drop in systolic pressure	5 Failure > 20 point drop in systolic pressure

18. Paradoxical Pupillary Reflex Test

Date	Score

1 Normal Pupil holds	2 Fair Holds but pulses after 10 secs.	3 Poor Pulses, becomes large after 10 secs.	4 Worse Pupil pulses, becomes large after 5 secs.	5 Failure Pupil immediately becomes large

NOTES:

Instructions for Performing In-Office Lab Tests

SALIVARY PH- STATIC MEASUREMENT

Testing must be done at least 30 minutes from any food or beverage.

1. Simply place a pH testing strip in the patient's mouth on top of the tongue and ask them to get it good and moist.

2. Lips must remain closed, as clinical readings of salivary pH must not allow exposure of the sample to air, which permits CO_2 loss, resulting in an inaccurate, increased pH reading.

3. Immediately after removing the pH strip (reading must be made within 3 seconds) compare the strip with the color code on the box.

DR. BIELER'S SALIVARY PH ACID CHALLENGE TEST

1. Cut seven 2" strips of pH paper and lay out on paper towel

2. Prepare lemon juice drink: 1 tablespoon of lemon juice and 1 tablespoon of water

3. Have patient make a pool of saliva in mouth and dip half of the strip, remove and measure pH. Record as baseline

4. Have patient drink lemon juice, check pH and start timing

Test and record pH every minute for 5 minutes

ZINC TASTE TEST

1. Patient's mouth should be free of any strong tastes

2. Patient holds 2 tablespoons of aqueous zinc in their mouth, sloshing it through the mouth

3. Start timing and have patient indicate when they taste the solution

4. Have them swallow

5. Ask them to describe the taste

Record strength of taste and seconds it took to taste the solution on the **Functional Terrain Analysis Form**

NOTES:

DR. KANE'S MINERAL ASSESSMENT TEST

1. Patient's mouth should be free of any strong tastes

2. Pour a small amount of liquid in bottle # 1 into a small cup

3. Patient holds the solution in their mouth, sloshing it around their mouth

4. Patient notes the taste, if any, of the solution. Use the forms that come with the test to accurately document each response.

5. Continue with the other solutions.

6. Record strength of taste for each solution on the **Functional Terrain Analysis Form**

URINE SPECIFIC GRAVITY USING A HYDROMETER

1. Fill urinometer with urine

2. Spin hydrometer in the urine

3. With hydrometer at eye level, read the specific gravity on the hydrometer by reading the bottom of the meniscus.

URINE PH USING PH METER

1. Remove protective cap on pH meter

2. Insert pH meter into urine specimen

3. Record digital reading

4. Clean pH meter

5. Calibration should take place after every 10-15 tests

URINARY ADRENAL TEST FOR URINARY CHLORIDE

1. Put 10 drops of urine into a small glass vial.

2. Add 1 drop of 20% Potassium Chromate—shake to mix.

3. Add <u>2.9%</u> Silver Nitrate, one drop at a time—shake to mix.

4. Record the number of drops it takes to produce a deep brick red color—no yellow remaining.

URINE CALCIUM TEST

1. Put a dropper full of urine into a disposable glass test tube

NOTES:

2.   Add one dropper of Sulkowitch Reagent- shake to mix

3.   Wait 60 seconds

4.   Observe turbidity:

        Record **CLEAR**…. if there is little to no discernible fine white precipitate

        Record **LIGHT**…. if you can see and read black type on a whit page through the vial

        Record **NORMAL**…. if the black type can be seen but not read through the vial

        Record **HEAVY**… if the black type cannot be seen through the vial and precipitate rolls in the liquid

        Record **MILKY**…. if it looks like milk which has been diluted with water

URINE SEDIMENT TEST

To determine the Total Urine Sediment:

CAUTION: Ferric Nitrate will stain yellow. Avoid contact with eyes, skin and clothing

1.   Add 10 ml of urine to a 15ml graduated centrifuge tube

2.   Add 4 drops of **50% Ferric Nitrate** solution. DO NOT shake or mix

3.   Centrifuge the tube for 30 seconds

4.   Pour off the fluid away from the plug of solid matter.

5.   Use the wooden end of a cotton applicator stick to level the sediment in the centrifuge tube.

6.   Measure the amount (volume) of sediment in ml by visualizing where the sediment would level out rather than averaging the high and low points

7.   Record as **total volume of the sediment** on the **Functional Terrain Analysis Form**

To determine sediment content:

Calcium phosphate sediment:

1.   Add enough **10% Acetic Acid** to equal the amount of sediment—shake or stir.

2.   Fill to 10 ml with Distilled Water.

3.   Centrifuge tube at 3400 rpm for 30 seconds.

4.   If sediment completely dissolves, record 100% **Calcium Phosphate**.

NOTES:

5. If sediment does not completely dissolve, pour off the fluid.

6. Measure the remaining sediment.

7. Subtract the remaining sediment measurement from the total sediment recorded above and record this number (in ml) as **Calcium Phosphate** on the **Functional Terrain Analysis Form**

Total sediment – remaining sediment = Calcium phosphate

Uric Acid Sediment:

1. Add enough **10% Sodium Hydroxide** to equal the amount of sediment remaining in the test tube—stir well until color turns red.

2. Fill to 10 ml with Distilled Water.

3. Centrifuge the tube for 30 seconds.

4. If sediment completely dissolves—record **Uric Acid** as the last amount (in ml) of sediment.

5. If sediment does not completely dissolve, pour off the fluid.

6. Measure the remaining sediment.

7. Subtract the remaining sediment from the previous remaining sediment calculated above and record this number (in ml) as **Uric Acid** on the **Functional Terrain Assessment Form**

Calcium Oxalate sediment:

Record the sediment remaining in the test tube as **Calcium Oxalate** on the **Functional Terrain Analysis Form**

OXIDATA FREE RADICAL TEST

1. Draw urine into the dropper supplied with the test kit

2. Break open the top of the glass ampoule, which contains the reagent

3. Place urine into the ampoule

4. Wait five minutes, then interpret the color change from the chart and record the result

NOTES:

BOWEL TOXICITY TEST FOR URINARY INDICAN

NOTE: Obermeyer's reagent is a strong acid that will cause burns. Wear safety goggles, rubber gloves and protective clothing. Please store away from metal objects, such as metal hinges on storage cabinets as it will corrode them!

1. Pour 5ml of urine into a 15ml graduated test tube

2. Add 5ml of Obermeyer's reagent

3. Seal the centrifuge with parafilm, hold in place with thumb and completely INVERT the tube 8 times to mix

4. Let the test tube sit for at least 5 minutes or until cool

5. Remove parafilm and add 2 ml of chloroform

6. Place a finger cot on a thumb and mix solution by inverting 8 times

7. Allow the chloroform to settle to the bottom.

8. Examine the color in the chloroform layer. A blue color indicates the presence of indican.

9. If the chloroform remains colorless, record "Zero" in the urinalysis report form.

10. If chloroform is blue add the saturated potassium chlorate solution, a drop at a time, mixing twice after each addition, and record the number of drops necessary to decolorize the chloroform.

11. Record the number of drops of potassium chlorate used to decolorize the blue in the **Functional Terrain Assessment Form**.

IODINE PATCH

1. Paint a 2 inch square patch of 2% solution of iodine onto the patient's abdomen

2. Make sure it is dry before allowing it to come in contact with clothing, because it will stain

3. Note the time of application and have patient record the time when they notice that it has disappeared

NOTES:

GASTROTEST FOR DETERMINING STOMACH pH

1. Have patient eat a protein rich meal 2 hours before test.

2. For an ambient pH have patient fast for 8-10 hours.

3. Get patient to swallow a little water to lubricate the throat

4. Swallow the capsule with a little water while the free end is held firmly outside the mouth

5. After capsule has been swallowed patient lies on left side or back on the table for 10 minutes.

6. After 10 minutes get the patient to sit up and with chin raised swiftly remove the string.

7. Lay string on paper and while the string is still moist touch the pH stick to the string starting at the distal end

8. The resultant colors are compared with the pH chart

NOTES:

CPT CODES AND SUGGESTED PRICES FOR IN-OFFICE LABORATORY TESTING

CPT	TEST	PRICE
86900	ABO blood typing	15
91052	Gastric analysis	20
82950	Glucose- blood	10
93720	Plethysmography, total body (body fat analysis)	30
83105	Hair analysis	See lab
83986	Salivary pH	10
81002	Urinalysis (dipstick)	15
82340	Urinary Calcium	10
82436	Urine Chloride (Urine Adrenal Test)	10
81099	Urine Indican (Bowel Toxicity Test)	10
81003	Urine pH	10
81099	Urinalysis panel (all terrain urinalysis tests)	65

NOTE: These codes are constantly being updated and changed. It is beyond the scope of this book to provide a full list of all available CPT codes. Please refer to your insurance manuals for more details.

The code 81099 is for any test using urine that has not been identified by a separate code.

NOTES:

PATIENT INFORMATION & INSTRUCTIONS FOR IN-OFFICE LAB TESTING

You have been scheduled for a series of in-office lab tests on: _____. These are laboratory tests performed in our office that will be providing valuable information about the underlying biochemistry and physiology of your body. It will help us identify and evaluate the areas of your body that are not functioning well. These simple tests analyze urine and saliva and other parameters to provide data on the acid-alkaline balance, and mineral, digestive, adrenal, and oxidative systems. In order to assure accurate results from this series of tests, it is very important for you to follow the instructions below:

3 days prior to the terrain test:
Please refrain from taking the following:
- Antacids
- Vitamins
- Minerals
- Enzymes.
- Other supplements

It is important to see how the body is coping without medications and supplements. Obviously, please continue with life essential medications.
Please also restrict your intake of salt i.e. do not salt the food on your plate

On the day of the terrain test:
9. On the morning of your test, obtain a sample of your **first** morning urine. Try to obtain a mid-stream specimen (urinate a small amount first, then obtain the remaining urine in your specimen cup). If a specimen cup did not reach you in time for your test, thoroughly wash a glass jar and lid (in the dishwasher is best) and use that instead. Some individuals may have to get up during the night or early morning to urinate. If this happens to you at 4:00 a.m. or later, collect this urine in your specimen cup. **Please refrigerate your sample.**
10. Please bring in today's **second** morning urine sample taken at least 1 hour later than your first morning sample. Please follow the instructions above for obtaining a mid-stream specimen in a clean specimen cup. **Again, please refrigerate sample**
11. Please bring a prescription list in with you if you had to take any life essential medications.
12. It is very important that you do not change your oral chemistry prior to the salivary testing. Please do not use the following for 1 hour before your scheduled appointment time for testing:
    13. Any food or drink
    14. Toothpaste
    15. Mouth wash
    16. Chewing gum
    17. Tobacco
    18. Dental prosthesis cleaner
19. Once the terrain testing has been run additional diagnostic tests may be performed in the office.

Thank you for your time and patience.

We look forward to working with you.

NOTES:

RESOURCES FOR IN OFFICE TESTING

A number of the tests mentioned in this book require you to purchase inexpensive kits or reagents. The following lists some of the suppliers of these resources.

Gastro Test

The Gastro-Test is manufactured in the US by HDC Corporation.

Mailing Address	Telephone	Web
628 Gibraltar Court, Milpitas, CA 95035	800-227-8162	http://www.hdccorp.com

Kanes Mineral Assessment Tests

The Kane Mineral Assessment Tests are manufactured in the US by E-Lyte, Inc.

Mailing Address	Telephone & Fax	Web
45 Reese Road Millville, NJ 08332	888-320-8338 (in US) 856-825-8338 (outside the US) Fax:856-852-2143	http://www.e-lyte.com

NOTES:

Oxidata Test

The Oxidata test is manufactured in the US by Apex.

Mailing Address	Telephone & Fax	Web
1701 E. Edinger Ave, Suite A-4, Santa Ana, CA 92705	714-973-7733 800-736-4381 Fax: 714-973-2238	www.oxidata.com www.apexenergetics.com

Apex Energetics also retails salivary pH paper and urine dipstick kits (Chemstrip 10)

Zinc Taste Test

The Zinc Taste test we recommend is manufactured in the US by Biotics Research Corporation.

Mailing Address	Telephone & Fax	Web
6801 Biotics Research Drive, Rosenberg, TX 77471	800-231-5777 Fax: 281-344-07725	www.BioticsResearch.com

United Kingdom

Mailing Address	Telephone	Web
Nutri-Link, Ltd. Nutrition House, 24 Torquay Road, Newton Abbott, Devon, TQ12 1AJ	01626 205417 Fax: 01626 205418	www.nutri-linkltd.co.uk/

NOTES:

<u>Urine reagents needed to do the Functional Urinalysis Testing</u>

Reagent	Amount
Chemstrips (100)	100 test strips
Obermeyer's reagent	16 ounce bottle
Chloroform	16 ounce bottle with 4 ounce decant bottle
Potassium chlorate	2 ounce bottle
Ferric nitrate	2 ounce bottle
Acetic acid	2 ounce bottle
Sodium hydroxide	2 ounce bottle
Potassium chromate	1 ounce bottle
Silver nitrate	2 ounce bottle
Sulkowitch reagent	4 ounce bottle

NOTE: Obermeyer's reagent contains hydrochloric acid, which can corrode metal. Please store away from any metal objects especially hinges on storage cabinets!

The above reagents can be ordered from the following company:

Rocky Mountain Reagents Inc
3207 West Hampden Avenue, Englewood, CO 80110
(303) 762-0800
www.rmreagents.com

They may require a copy of your professional license.

NOTES:

SETTING UP AN IN-OFFICE LAB

The following section explains how to set up an in-office lab, and provides you with a list of the materials, reagents, and testing supplies you will need to set up a functional in-office lab testing facility in your clinic. You do not need a lot of space to set up a functional lab in your clinic. I used to run the tests in a small bathroom when I first started running this battery of tests on my patients. The space must be well ventilated, well lit, and have running water.

This is a photo of what equipment you will need:

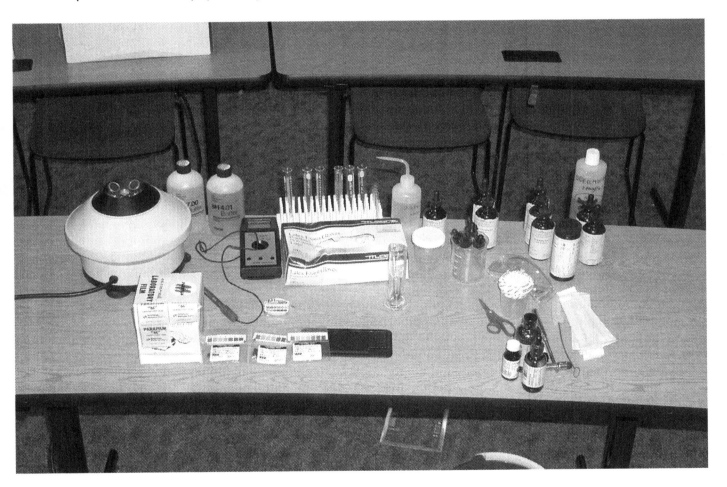

NOTES:

What to include in your In-Office testing Kit

Equipment	Quantity Needed
Centrifuge	1
pH Meter	1
Finger cots	1 box
Test tubes (box of 250)	1 box
Applicator sticks (box of 1000)	100 individual applicator sticks
Safety glasses	1
Urinometer (float and jar)	1
Graduated cylinders	4
Graduated cylinder brush	1
Test tube racks	1
Wash bottles	1
Funnels	1
Glass droppers	6
Beakers	2
Parafilm	1 box
Iodine patch test	1 bottle
Zinc tally	1 bottle
PH paper	1 roll
Dr. Kane's mineral assessment tests	1 test kit
Gastro string test	5 tests
Oral Thermometers	5 to loan to patients

NOTES:

A few words of caution about Obermeyer's reagent and the Bowel Toxicty Test:

- Do not pour the reagents from the Bowel Toxicity Test down your sink. The acid in the Obermeyer's reagent will quickly damage your plumbing. I suggest that you pour the reagents into the bowl of your toilet and flush.

- You do not need a hooded vent to do the Bowel toxicity test. I highly recommend safety glasses, and of course gloves. Do this test in a well ventilated space, preferably with a extraction fan.

- Do not store your Obermeyer's reagent in a cabinet with metal hinges. The acid in the reagent can corrode the metal hinges over time. I found out about this the hard way!

Places to obtain In-Office Lab Equipment:

Centrifuge: You can buy one from second hand medical suppliers or get one from your blood testing lab.

pH Meter: The best bet is to search on the internet. Hanna instruments make a very reasonable pH meter, which is ideal for doing accurate pH measurements on Urine.

Test tubes, finger cots etc.: Rocky Mountain Reagents is a one-stop resource for all of the equipment you need to set up a Functional In-Office Lab. Their address and phone number are:

Rocky Mountain Reagents Inc
3207 West Hampden Avenue, Englewood, CO 80110
(303) 762-0800
www.rmreagents.com

You may also want to try a medical supply company. The one I have used is:

Moore Medical
1-800-234-1464
Fax: 1-800-944-6667

All of the forms in this book are available as master copies to be used in your clinic. They are free of charge.

Please visit:

http://www.BloodChemistryAnalysis.com/urinalysis-downloads.html

BIBLIOGRAPHY

Loomis, H., Physical and Laboratory Identification of Enzyme Deficiencies, 21st Century Enzyme Inc., 1990

Fischbach, F., A manual of Laboratory and Diagnostic Tests, 5th edition, Lippincott, 1996

Great Smokies Diagnostic laboratory, Functional assessment resource manual, 1999

Marz, R., Medical Nutrition from Marz, 2nd edition, Omni-press 1997

DeGowin, R.L., DeGowin and De Gowin's Diagnostic Examination, 6th edition, McGraw Hill, 1994

Sherman, J. et al., 24 Hour Urine Assay A dynamic interpretation of Cellular Function, NCNM 1990

Diagnos-Tech, Inc., Adrenal Stress Index Salivary Testing, 1998

Schenker, G.R., An Analytical System of Clinical Nutrition, 2nd edition, 1995

The "Four Quadrants of Functional Diagnosis"
Diagnostic Education for the *Functional Age*

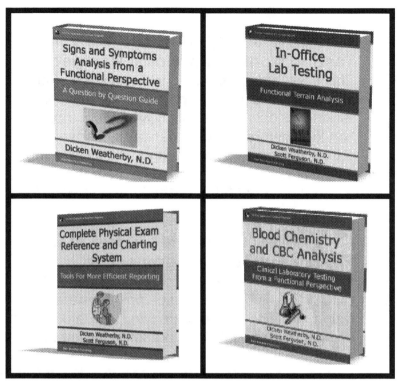

Most of us at some point or other have come to recognize that the diagnostic tests we learned in medical school taught us nothing about how to uncover our patients' functional problems. This is why I wrote my first book, *"Blood Chemistry and CBC Analysis- Clinical Laboratory Testing From a Functional Perspective"* with my colleague Dr. Scott Ferguson, to make the wealth of functional information you can get from a standard Chemistry Screen and CBC available to health care practitioners. This book and other products in my "Four Quadrants of Functional Diagnosis" series are designed to give you and your practice the same functional diagnostic education that thousands of practitioners have been using successfully in their practices.

The *Four Quadrants of Functional Diagnosis* will help you:
- Get excellent patient results
- Dramatically improve your clinical outcomes
- Get more referrals
- Cut the amount of time you spend analyzing your patient cases
- Set up a system of functional tests that will be the envy of all your colleagues

In preparing for the Functional Age, the rules on how to manage the diagnostic information in your practice have changed. You can no longer blindly use the same tests every one else is using and hope to get different results. The Functional Age will require that you have more information to be able to properly find the cause of your patients' problems. *Signs and Symptoms Analysis from A Functional Perspective, Boost Clinic Income With an In-Office Lab System,* and *The Functional Blood Chemistry Analysis System* were developed for practitioners just like you who recognize the need for a new paradigm in diagnostic information. Practitioners who realize that the Pathological Age is over and the Functional Age has begun.

Dr. Dicken Weatherby, Naturopathic Physician

Functional Blood Chemistry Analysis

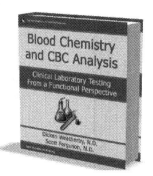

Blood Chemistry and CBC Analysis- Clinical Laboratory Testing from a Functional Perspective

This book presents a diagnostic system of blood chemistry and CBC analysis that focuses on physiological function as a marker of health. By looking for optimum function we increase our ability to detect dysfunction long before disease manifests. Conventional lab testing becomes a truly preventative and prognostic tool. A must for any practitioners who wants to get more from the tests they are already running.
Printed Book $65.00 (in the U.S.A.) ISBN: 0-9761367-1-6

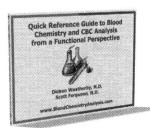

Quick Reference Guide to Blood Chemistry Analysis From a Functional Perspective

This guide is the perfect companion to our Blood Chemistry and CBC Analysis Book. It is a complete reference for interpreting, analyzing, and finding the underlying cause of your patients' functional complaints. You will find yourself referring to this guide over and over again.
Printed Book $35.00 (in the U.S.A.) ISBN: 0-9761367-8-3

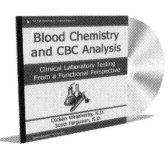

Functional Blood Chemistry Analysis Seminar on Audio

Any practitioners of the healing arts will gain a tremendous benefit from listening to this complete one day seminar on audio CD. Dr. Weatherby guides the listener through his method of analyzing blood chemistry and CBC tests. Topics include using standard blood tests to analyze the following: GI dysfunction, minerals and vitamin insufficiencies, blood sugar dysregulation, cardiovascular problems, thyroid issues, and adrenal dysfunction..
6 hours of audio $147.00 (in the U.S.A.) ISBN: 0-9726469-4-9

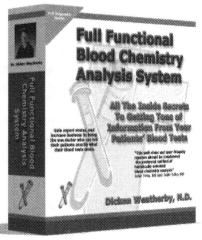

The Full Functional Blood Chemistry Analysis System is a complete road map to success that shows you exactly how to approach each blood chemistry analysis step by step. This system includes the printed reference book, the Quick Reference Guide, and the Audio Recordings, a system for getting the most out of your blood chemistry tests.

A functional diagnosis of your patients' blood test results is one of the most effective diagnostic tools to get to the bottom of the myriad of health complaints your patients present with. Gain expert status, and increase business by being the one doctor who can tell patients exactly what their blood tests mean.
Full Blood Chemistry System $197.00 (in the U.S.A.) ISBN: 0-9761367-3-2

In-Office Lab Testing
Boost Your Clinic Income!

I want you to be successful in your practice and to have the same tools that I use to increase clinical efficacy and clinic income, which is why I created my *Boost Clinic Income With an In-Office Lab System.* The tests I present in this system will help you get a wealth of functional data from your patients and the income you make on these tests stays in your practice. At the heart of this system is my Functional Urinalysis program.

Functional Urinalysis allows you to run a series of simple urine tests that get to the heart of the disturbances in your patients' inner "terrain". These tests have been used for many years but until now the interpretive information available to health care practitioners has been poor. I have put together the most comprehensive system for understanding and interpreting the Functional Urinalysis. Watch the instructional DVD, listen to the 2 audio CDs packed with time saving tips and interpretive tools, refer to the in-depth reference manual, and start paying for your office overhead with Functional Urinalysis!

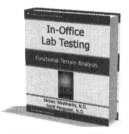
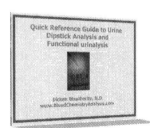
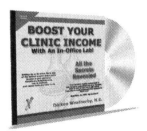
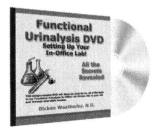
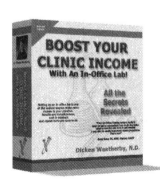

Other Functional Diagnostic Tools

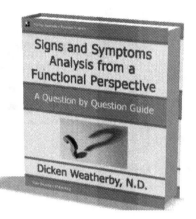

Signs and Symptoms Analysis From a Functional Perspective

This book takes a critical look at the myriad of signs and symptoms a patient presents with. Using a comprehensive signs and symptoms questionnaire you can look at the symptom burden in specific systems of the body, address some of the more obscure symptoms, and track changes over time. Organized by body systems, this book provides the nutritional and functional explanations behind the 322 questions on Dr. Weatherby's 4-page questionnaire.

Printed Book $65.00 (in the U.S.A.) ISBN: 0-9761367-2-4

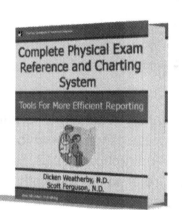

Complete PE Reference and Charting System

Drs. Weatherby and Ferguson have put together report forms for all the major physical examinations commonly performed in your office (i.e. cardiovascular, lung, abdominal, neurological examinations). These report forms provide an easy method of charting and filing your physical examination results.

The accompanying reference cards fit neatly into your white coat and provide a detailed explanation of all the tests on each report form and are an excellent "exam-side" reference to refresh your memory on all the different tests that make up each examination.

Printed Reference Cards and CD $65.00 (in the U.S.A.)

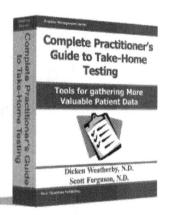

Complete Practitioner's Guide to Take-Home Testing

Drs. Weatherby and Ferguson have put together a series of 17 take-home tests that you can give to your patients to perform in between their office visits. These tests will allow you to assess for digestion, elimination, zinc status, pH regulation, hypothyroid conditions, iodine insufficiency, blood type, and food and other sensitivities and intolerances. Patient "homework" is an important method of gathering patient data and encouraging compliance.

Printed Book $45.00 (in the U.S.A.) ISBN: 0-9761367-7-5

Quick Order Form

Fax Orders: 541-488-0323. Send this form.

Telephone orders: Call 541-482-3779

Email orders: orders@bBloodChemistryAnalysis.com

Secure online orders: http://www.BloodChemistryAnalysis.com/diagnosisshop.html

Postal orders: Weatherby & Associates, LLC, 2693 Takelma Way, Ashland, OR 97520, USA. Telephone: 541-482-3779

Please send the following books, CDs or reports. I understand that I may return any of them for a full refund – for any reason, no questions asked.

_____
_____
_____

Please send more FREE information on:

☐ Other books ☐ Live Seminars or Teleseminars ☐ Speaking ☐ Consulting

Name:_____

Address:_____

City:_____ State: _____ Zip:_____

Phone:_____ E-mail:_____

Shipping by air
US: $4.00 for first book and $2.00 for each additional product.
International: $9.00 for first book; $5.00 for each additional product (estimate)

Payment: ☐ Cheque   ☐ Credit Card
☐ Visa   ☐ Mastercard   ☐ AMEX   ☐ Discover

Personal check (payable to Weatherby & Associates, LLC):

Card number:_____

Name on card:_____Exp. Date:_____

http://www.BloodChemistryAnalysis.com

Printed in the USA
CPSIA information can be obtained
at www.ICGtesting.com
LVHW010735301023
762524LV00010B/136